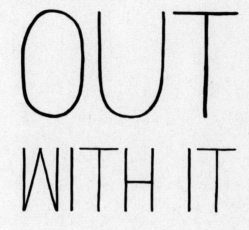

OUT
WITH IT

OUT
WITH IT

HOW STUTTERING
HELPED ME FIND MY VOICE

Katherine Preston

ATRIA BOOKS
New York • London • Toronto • Sydney • New Delhi

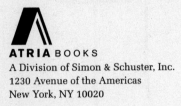 ATRIA BOOKS

A Division of Simon & Schuster, Inc.
1230 Avenue of the Americas
New York, NY 10020

First Atria Books hardcover edition April 2013

ATRIA BOOKS and colophon are trademarks of Simon & Schuster, Inc.

For information about special discounts for bulk purchases,
please contact Simon & Schuster Special Sales at 1-866-506-1949
or business@simonandschuster.com.

The Simon & Schuster Speakers Bureau can bring authors to your
live event. For more information or to book an event, contact the
Simon & Schuster Speakers Bureau at 1-866-248-3049 or visit our
website at www.simonspeakers.com.

Designed by Dana Sloan

Manufactured in the United States of America

10 9 8 7 6 5 4 3 2 1

Library of Congress Cataloging-in-Publication Data

Preston, Katherine, date.
    Out with it : how stuttering helped me find my voice / Katherine
Preston. — First Atria Books hardcover edition.
        pages cm
    1. Preston, Katherine, date—Health. 2. Stutterers—Biography.
3. Stutterers—Rehabilitation. I. Title.
    RC424.P932 2013
    616.85'540092—dc23
    [B]   2012048984

ISBN 978-1-4516-7658-7
ISBN 978-1-4516-7660-0 (ebook)

For my parents, with much love

CONTENTS

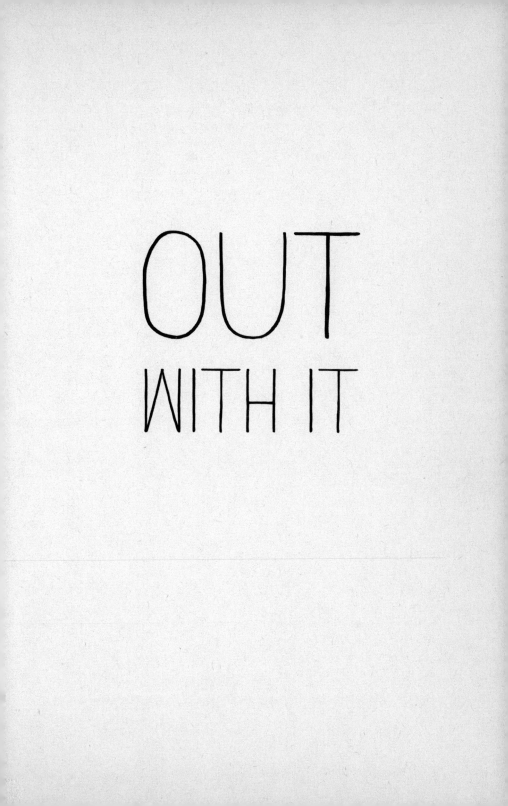

OUT
WITH IT

PROLOGUE

I CAN TASTE THE other side of my name, and yet it hangs resolutely out of reach. The wall has come down. My name has been broken in half. My tongue lies taut and heavy, the tip glued to the base of my mouth.

"KKKKK KK K K K K K K. K K K K K KK kkkkkkk kaaa kaa."

I feel the familiar hand clench slowly around my throat. As the seconds pass, my chest twists tighter. Panic winds its way through my nervous system and holds my useless body hostage.

"KK kkkk kkk kaaa ka ka."

My fingernails dig into my palms in penance. My knees lock my legs and freeze my body into position. My eyes widen desperately. I can taste the stale air as it slips out of my mouth. I have no idea if I will say the word or if I will be trapped here indefinitely.

Desperate, unfocused anger addles my brain and pricks at my pores. I hate the boy's intrusion, I hate his cocky swagger

1

and his half-cocked head. I hate the fact that my parents aren't here to pick me up, I hate the stupid party and my stupid outfit. I hate everything and nothing. Because I can't hate my stutter; I can't shout at my stutter to vent my frustration.

As the sound of my name falters onwards, my thoughts wander further. Why did I even answer him? Why did I not just plead temporary deafness? I knew that I would stutter. I am ten years old and have been doing it spectacularly for the past three years. My name is the one word that never escapes my mouth unscathed.

But somehow I had lost my memory in the past couple of hours. I had forgotten that I was a stutterer, or forgotten that I should be scared of stuttering. We had been at a birthday party, and I was leaving the house basking in the glow of a slightly nauseous sugar rush. I was dragging a deflated balloon from my wrist, looking to see where Claire had gone, when the boy called out to ask my name. I recognized his face from the room and responded more out of politeness than anything else.

Thirty seconds have ticked by and I'm tired. I'm tired at the thought of speaking and tired by the breathless, unresolved end of my past expulsion. I wish I was home, wish I was anywhere but here on this stretch of endless gray pavement. My inquisitor is confused, and I hope that I can still recover. I force myself to believe that this time will be different. Like a madman, I pray for the same action to have a new outcome. I take a deep breath and run up at the word again.

"K K K K K K Kaaaa Kaaa . . ."

I watch confusion morph into mirth. I have really blown

it now. I can almost hear the question forming in his brain as he smirks at me,

"What the hell?" He says it slowly and then breaks into giggles, "Did you forget your name?"

His face cracks open in glee. He waves at his friends dispersing out down the road. They look bored, and his raucous laughter promises its normal level of fabulous entertainment. They start wandering back to him.

"Tell us all your name."

I am trapped and I know it. My options are: (a) refuse to say my name and be forced to face clever insults like "retard," or (b) stutter. Neither fills me with joy. I flick my head round quickly. I can see Claire now. She's striding down the road, at least five cars away. Her parents are waiting for us. I'm alone.

"What's wrong? Cat got your tongue?"

I imagine myself asking him what exactly that phrase means. I have recently learnt the word *cliché* and picture myself silencing his taunts and leading us all into a friendly discussion on some of the crazier phrases we have heard people say. Sadly, my reality is a little less rosy. His friends are gathering now, and all five freshly scrubbed faces are staring at me.

"What are you looking at?" my bitter voice pipes up from nowhere. As clearly as I knew I couldn't say my name, I knew that the nervous energy would propel my voice, allow me to utter something. I have learnt from bitter experience that anger makes me fluent, that I could be just like the rest of the world if only I would shout every question and swear my way through every answer.

Briefly, my question silences them. My accent is English, home counties, girly, nothing fabulously interesting. They look up at their ringleader. I suspect that they are wondering why he has called them over. They clearly have more important business to attend to, and two of them wander off, bored.

I relax for a moment, but the boy keeps staring at me. I feel like a monkey on a chain. I have not performed how he was hoping. He looks vaguely put out. His humiliation swells in front of me and billows out onto his ruddy cheeks. I try to walk away, my head held high and haughty, but something holds me to the cement. I have tasted fluency and now want to prove him wrong. I want to make him feel small.

Then, suddenly, it looks like he has realized something. I didn't say my name. I see it cross his eyes, a flicker of hope. He has seen how he can redeem himself to the two remaining members of his fan club.

"Tell these guys your name," he sneers at me.

"Why should I?"

Damn, why did I say that? Now he knows he has me. I have to do it now. Now they're all looking at me.

The thing is, I know I'll stutter. On my name I have no chance. And I desperately want to keep my dignity. A girl does not get dressed up in orange leggings and an oversized tie-dye T-shirt to lose her self-respect to a bunch of scruffy boys with no sense of style.

So I pull myself up to my full height. All four feet two inches of me stares up at them.

"K . . ."

"Katherine, Katherine Preston. And what's it to you?" she practically spits at them. Claire stops and takes a replenishing breath. "Why do you even care? Why don't you go and talk to your own friends, or are you that unpopular that you need to hassle girls who aren't remotely interested in talking to you?"

She's on a roll. Inwardly, relief splashes across my body. Her face is flushed from running back to me. There are now two of us. Two leggings-clad, vertically challenged warriors.

"I'm sure you have nothing better to do, but we have better places to be than wasting our time talking to you."

She slips her arm through mine and we turn on the balls of our feet in unison. We swing away from them and march triumphantly down the road.

"Thank you," I whisper.

She is still striding, all fierce and self-righteous. "God, I hate boys."

"Me, too."

We leave it at that. I pray that it will be the last time we will speak of it. I suspect it will. If we never mention it again, maybe she will forget about it and maybe I will.

She seems to forget almost instantly, but I can't push it aside as quickly as I'd like. I sit in the backseat of her parents' car and stare out at the familiar scenes of London as Claire tells them all about the party. As we drive down the embankment, along the dark stretch of the Thames, I replay the smirk on the boy's face. As we drive past the familiar brick houses, I can still feel the fear lick around my insides. I can't ignore the fact that I have been saved, that I can't save myself. As absurdly grateful as I am to Claire, I feel pathetic. What kind of a kid can't stick up for herself? What will I do the next time? What will I do if I am on my own?

That night I sit on the bottom bunk of my bed and address our new Labrador puppy. She is meant to be downstairs in the kitchen, but I have smuggled her up to my room. I suspect that we are both a little lonely. I am an only child and, as quiet as it can be at times, there are moments when it has its benefits. Right now, I'm grateful there's no sister on the top bunk, no brother down the hall. Claire has been my best friend since I was four years old. She has barely been out of my sight in six years, but right now I can't bear the thought of her company. I can't stomach the idea of any company at all. Except Holly. Being a dog, Holly doesn't count. I am certain that I'll be fluent around her.

I have never stuttered in a room on my own, and I have never stuttered in front of an animal. I have always known what my fluent voice sounds like, have always known that it exists somewhere inside of me.

"Why am I such a stumbling wreck when I talk to people?" I whisper to Holly.

The quiet sound of my voice gives me some solace. It is comforting to hear that I'm not entirely broken, that I still have a voice, however meager it can sound at times.

"What's wrong with me?"

Holly looks up, wags her tail, does a couple of laps on my bed, and then lies down looking at me. I grab the rope toy that I have brought up with me and watch her chase it manically for a few moments. She grabs hold and tugs until I let go. I watch her nudge it back towards me.

I wipe a couple of traitorous tears from my cheek. "I know, I know, you think I'm alright," I don't want Holly to think I am pathetic. She is under my care; I feel that I have someone else to look after for the first time in my life. I'm not keen to let her down and I want to keep her loyalty.

"But some people think I'm weird, a freak." I am gulping a little as I watch her cock her head. She moves towards the side of the bed and, not wanting to let go of her warmth, I pull her into my lap and add, "Don't worry—it's mostly smelly boys." I'm not sure who I'm trying to reassure.

"Why do I have to talk funny?" I nuzzle my forehead against the soft golden fuzz of her head and ruffle her ears until she starts to squirm in my arms. As I lift her to face me, I have stopped sniffling, "You know, if I was fluent, I could be an actress. Or a TV presenter. I would tell everyone everything that was on my mind. I'd be eloquent and witty and insightful. You would never be able to shut me up. I would enter competitions for people who could talk the most."

She manages to wriggle free, jumps off the bed, and starts turning circles by the door. I lift her into the nook of my waist and, as silently as possible, creak my bedroom door open. I have to keep it quiet; the last thing I want to do is wake my parents. I creep out of my room and carry her squirming body back down the stairs to the kitchen. As I stretch my legs over the steps that I know will creak, I can see the boxes spilling out of various rooms. I can see my teddies breaking free of one cardboard box and our old photo albums sneaking out of another. I notice that my dad's golf clubs are stacked up by the front door.

We are moving house, leaving our Knightsbridge town house and moving to a house far, far away in the countryside. For months I had begged my parents to leave London. I had presented my arguments relentlessly over days and weeks, slowly chipping away at their hesitancy. I had listed the benefits of living in the country: the cleaner air, the fields to run around in, the possibility of having a bigger home, the room to breathe. They had stalled, spoken to friends, whispered their conversations late into the night. Finally, they had agreed; we would give it a go, see if we liked it.

I had been ecstatic when they told me. Now I'm a little more nervous. Will it work? As I put Holly back into her bed, I whisper that she'll love our new home, there will be hundreds of pheasants for her to chase all day. I promise her that, as much as I hate change, I think this is a good change, I hope it is. I reassure her that we are heading to a new place, a new beginning.

The discoloration on the wall next to her head catches my eye. I doubt that anyone else would see it, but I know it is there, however well disguised. I stare at the lick of fresh white paint and brush my fingers against the fine hairs of the brushstrokes. It is a guilty reminder of all the mornings that we have come down to find a pile of rubble under Holly's tiny paws. A sad testament to all the nights she must have spent desperately tunneling into the brick wall of our kitchen.

I know that my dad has patiently filled in the holes every morning with plaster and taken out his paint pot before the real estate agent comes around with another prospective buyer to trample around our home. I have heard him joke with his friends that she's impressively strong for a three-month-old puppy, that one day the plaster may all fall out, and whoever ends up with the house will worry that they've been landed with the ghost of gigantic termites. I hope that tonight she'll stay asleep until the morning.

As I start to sneak back upstairs I resolve that this year will be different, that this year I will tackle my stutter once and for all. I will teach myself how to be the same as everyone else. I give myself a checklist:

1. Say my name very loudly out of my window ten times every evening.
2. Ask every stranger I meet on the street what the time is.
3. Take ten deep breaths every morning.
4. Watch how Mum speaks and talk like her.

Foolproof. I give myself just over six months. If I can speak fluently on my own, then surely I can make myself speak "properly" when I'm out in public. I tell myself that I'm just lazy, that I just have to try harder. Through force of will, I will make myself fluent by the age of eleven.

FOR MUCH of my childhood I made promises. I promised myself that I would change, that I would rid myself of my stutter. For much of my life I believed, unfairly, that it was simply a matter of willpower. Over the years I would watch myself fail at fluency, and every morning I would wake up with the dangerously impractical resolution that today would be different, that I would be stronger, that I would force my speech into submission. I stubbornly clung to the hope that one day I would wake up and the stutter would have simply disappeared.

When I was ten years old I was far too busy house-training my dog and trying to fit in at my new school, to make time in my day for getting comfortable in my own skin. I was far too focused on reaching for perfection and not at all interested in seeing the good in my unique speech patterns. I was obsessed with speech and desperate to get rid of my stutter.

Every second that I spoke seemed to drag into a year. Every tiny interaction felt like an obstacle course ready to trip me up. I had started to watch others with jealous interest, and I fiercely guarded any fluency that I chanced upon. Less than ten stutters a day was a good day, over a hundred was a very bad day indeed. I was a happy child, I had a largely idyllic life, I rarely felt sorry for myself. Yet I was what my mum termed a "worrywart." I was easily hurt, highly sensitive, and my emotions swung from intense joy to deep fear.

Having witnessed some of my struggles, my parents had tried to help. They had done their research and found the best speech therapists that London had to offer. They did anything they could, made any move they could, to make me feel secure and happy. Yet none of it was helping and, at ten years old, my misguided, self-taught attempts to find fluency began to feel like the only viable option. I had to succeed. If I didn't become fluent, I wasn't sure what would happen to me.

OUT WITH IT   **11**

At the crux of it all I was terrified. I was afraid of what people would think of me, afraid of suffocating on my still-born words, and afraid of the lack of control I had over my own speech. The terror crashed through my armor and made me desperate to fight.

For better or worse, I knew that I couldn't hide my stutter, however much I tried. I felt like I had been dealt a hand of low cards at a poker table. No one had taught me the rules, but folding wasn't an option, so I needed a strategy. I needed a way to either become normal or deal with not being normal. I didn't know of any role models for stutterers: Porky Pig was hardly a leader of men, and the odd stutterer that I came across in films was classed as the comedy buffoon. With no roadmap, I barreled forward the best way I could.

I repeated words, went red in the face, looked at the floor, gasped for breath, and employed a little light pinching when I couldn't expel a single sound. Stuttering was my "thing," it exposed me and marked me as different. I dreamed of being "normal" and relentlessly worried about my "abnormality."

But I wasn't alone. As we got older, some girls started to worry about their weight, some threw up after every meal, some had acne that scarred their faces and filled their cupboards with fearful-looking creams, some had small boobs, others had big boobs. Others ran razors over their arms, making the skin under their school shirts raw and jagged. Some had to deal with the confusing territory of their sexuality. As exams started to mark the years of our lives, some cried into their textbooks as large red Cs and Ds stained their pages, and they worried that they were suited only for a lifetime of menial labor. We all fought ourselves and worried about what would happen to us. We all struggled to get comfortable in our own skins. Or I assume we did. No one spoke about it. We were English, after all.

As I was growing up, I created this myth that if I worked to better myself every day, I would eventually reach some nirvana of perfection where all my problems would disappear. I thought that hiding my stutter, or somehow magically growing out of my hesitant speech, was the only option. I saw my speech as something to be ashamed of, something only I did, something born of common laziness.

If some Tarot card–wielding fortuneteller had told my younger self that one day stuttering would be the driving force in my life, that it would push me to leave my life in London and set off on a mission to interview hundreds of fellow stutterers, I would have rolled my eyes. Having believed that I was one of a small handful of stutterers, I wonder if I would have been appalled or comforted to find out that there were millions of us across the globe. I'm certain that I would have demanded my money back if she had told me that my research into stuttering would turn into a memoir, that, in telling the stories of the people I met, I would realize that I was unraveling my own story.

And yet, at the age of twenty-four, I did just that. I set off on the road to spend a year with people like me, people who had at one time been labeled "abnormal." I set off on a quest to interview everyone from celebrities to hermits in order to find out what sort of lives they had created for themselves. My stutter, and my barely acknowledged search for a cure, led me across a country I had dreamed of exploring and to a final resolution that I would have never expected. As much as this is my story, it belongs to every stutterer, parent, friend, therapist, and researcher who spoke to me. It is as much their story as it is mine; it is my tribute to their courage and their honesty.

Out With It is about all of us and all the ways that it matters to make ourselves heard. It is about struggling with a different voice and speaking up regardless. It is about working out what you need to say, and finding the courage to say it. It is an account of my confounding journey to get to grips with being a "stutterer," about all the underprepared and uninformed ways that I tackled coming to terms with myself. Most of it isn't pretty. I'm sure a handy guidebook would have been appreciated, but this is the story of how I finally found my voice.

PART ONE

ENGLAND

CHAPTER 1

CREATION MYTH

London, April 1991

I WAS SEVEN YEARS old when I lost my voice. It happened without the fanfare I would have hoped for. It just quietly slipped away one day while I was showing off my new ballet uniform.

I'm standing with my hands on my hips, one foot poised on the tip of my toes. The elastic of the cotton leotard nips in at my waist and clips uncomfortably between my legs. A pathetic attempt at a skirt reaches out, almost horizontally, in stiff layers of pink gauze. Looking at my figure in the mirror, I proudly appraise my cocooned white legs and the neat silk bows I have recently learnt to tie around my ankles. I pivot on my tiptoes and hurry out of my bedroom, keen to show my mum the birthday present she has given me. I slide and trip leaping down the carpeted stairs, landing ungracefully at my godmother's feet. "Look," I half-bellow, half-plead, as I rush to regain my ballerina's posture, "I look like Angelina bbb b b bbb b b bbb ballerina!"

In my mind I have magically morphed into a female mouse. I'm too taken with the idea to worry much about the stalling rhythm of my delivery. I can see the excitement on her face. But it is laced with something else, hesitancy perhaps.

Joey is one of mum's oldest friends. She tells the funniest jokes and dances the best at parties. Most important, she treats me like I'm an adult. She makes my list of top ten favorite people, and I can't stop myself from being desperate for her praise. She oohs and aahs as she hugs me but, as I start to tell her all about my dance classes and my latest teacher, I watch her initial hesitancy grow. The shadow of a frown sweeps across her normally beaming face.

I know that I have rushed my words together in the past, that I have a tendency to slip them into one another and barrel forward regardless. But I love to tell stories, love the interest of my parents' friends. Caught up in my own excitement, I have never paid much attention to other people's reactions. Had they always looked a bit surprised when I spoke? I guess that I may have seen the odd strange reaction, but I have definitely not paid it much notice before.

I wish I could do the same now, but suddenly it is hard not to notice Joey. She matters more to me than most people. I put my hands firmly on my hips and try again, "Will you be able to come to my next ba ba baaaaa." I run up to the broken word again. It's no good. I can't get past the *b*. It is trapped, locked beneath the barrier that has closed the path from my lungs to my mouth. I sound like the old, scratched Cat Stevens records that my dad sometimes plays. The strange clench has exposed a tear in my system, a gaping hole that I need to jump across. "Baaaa baba baaa ballet performance."

We look at each other for a long second. She is normally full of stories, but she is silent now, and the final expulsion of the word has left me slightly out of breath. She tells me that, of course she'll be there and leans over the banister to call down the stairs, "Janey." I wonder if I can hear a trace of nervousness in her voice: "Katherine has something she wants to show you." We stand there in silence. She smiles at me as the click of my mum's high heels on the kitchen floor signal that she is on her way. We hear her soft footsteps up the carpeted stairs, and then there she is, wiping her hands on a kitchen towel. "Wow, look at you, love. What a sight. When is your next lesson?"

"Its on M m m m m m m m m." The air locks in my throat again. This time my lips vibrate and my mouth is glued shut. For the first time I decide to push harder, I decide to push against the clamp that's tightening around my throat. I don't want to see her reaction, whatever it might be, so I look down at the floor. The air stagnates and then begins to slip slowly from my lungs. I begin to feel faint and woozy, I worry that I could somehow suffocate myself. The fear opens my eyes wide and disconnects me briefly from my body. On the last shred of breath my voice emerges, shattered into pieces, "m m m m m mmm mmon mon mon day."

I know that unintentionally I have done something very

wrong, something unnatural. I scuff my once-pristine shoes on the wooden banister. Seconds pass and then curiosity gets the better of me. Tentatively I look back up at her face.

She is crouching next to me, her face almost level with mine. I can hear her tell me how excited I must be for my upcoming class. Her bright smile calms me. I listen to her tell Joey what a good ballet dancer I am. I feel her thread her little finger through mine and ask me if I'll come downstairs and help her cook. As I make my way slowly down the stairs, I wonder if maybe I imagined everything before. I try to force the memory out of my head. Yet as she lifts me up onto the counter, I can't help but wonder what will happen the next time I open my mouth.

TODAY, LOOKING back, I question the reliability of my memory. I can clearly picture that day, and yet I wonder how much of it is remembered and how much is reconstructed from conversations and photos and restrained diary entries. I wonder if I have told myself the story so many times that the facts don't matter anymore, that the tale that I told myself, the day that we all thought we remembered, became part of my makeup. I wonder about all the other stories, all the stories that I heard from others who remember the first time they stuttered. I wonder if we all have half-remembered jigsaw pieces that we glue together and build into a cohesive narrative.

Over the years my convictions have been smudged because I have seen how we all like to find a reason for everything. We like to single out one moment to hinge the rest of our lives around, the tipping point when we slip from one reality to the next. Stuttering falls into that pattern almost too easily.

Nearly every stutterer has heard a family tale for why they stutter. Their stories become predictable when you have heard enough. Almost universally, they revolve around physical pain, emotional repression, illness, or death. Bobby Childers, a New Mexico computer technician, remembers climbing up a tree at his granddad's ranch as a young child. He remembers losing his grip and falling twenty feet until he hit the ground. "I started to cry, and my father and my granddad and my uncle came over and said, 'Men don't cry.' So I stopped crying, and I haven't cried since. I was told that within a few months I began stuttering. I don't know if that was the cause or not. That was just what I was told."

Speech therapist Eric Jackson now knows that in most cases stuttering begins when you start combining words, when you start talking, between the ages of two and three. However, for twenty-five years of his life, Eric believed something entirely different. His whole family traced his stutter back to the year that he had his tonsils taken out. "I was really sick and, for a few days afterwards, I had a 106-degree fever," he remembers. "I'm sure that there was talk of possible brain damage after being in a high fever for that long. So, for my entire life, up until that point, my parents told me that the reason I stuttered was because I got really sick when I was three years old."

We all have our own mythology, our personal moment that pinpoints the day our lives changed. Today I know that my own stutter didn't come out of thin air. As much as I once wanted a pivot, an event to make sense of it all, I now know that I was born with a stutter lurking deep within my system. A speech therapist report from two years earlier tells me that I was having difficulty with certain letters, and my mum remembers that I always spoke fast, galloping towards my point too quickly to piece my words together properly. I was an unusually outgoing child, and she assumed I was just eager to spit out my words.

In all likelihood, my stutter had been around for a while, and I hadn't thought much of it. But at seven years old, I began to see the way that people reacted to me, the confused expressions that I had not paid much attention to before. Plus, at seven years old, everyone paid a little more attention to my stumbling delivery, everyone worried a little more about my emotional stability. It was the year my grandma died.

She had come to live with us four months earlier. My parents had insisted, they had driven down to her little bungalow just south of London to pick her up. She had walked up the three floors to our guest bedroom, smiling and joking as she panted for breath, my parents on either side ready to catch her if she lost consciousness. As she sat on the edge of the double bed, her tiny frame seemed dwarfed by the room. As my parents went to get her bags, she held my hand and asked me to lift myself onto the bed next to her. I climbed up and told her stories about my day. I showed her my teddy, told her what he liked to eat, who he liked to spend time with. She nodded sagely and patiently asked serious questions about my other toys. As Mum and Dad hung up her clothes, I ran downstairs to get her some orange juice and climbed back up the stairs one at a time, to tell her how much fun we would have making forts out of her duvet and pillows.

I knew that she was ill, knew that it was serious, but I loved having her in the house. For the first two months, I rushed home from school to see her. I loved how she insisted that she eat with me before the sun set so my parents could eat on their own later. Gradually, she could no longer make the trek up and down the stairs and, ensconced in our guest room, her famous apple pie and her talent for Easter egg hunt riddles seemed to fade into rose-tinted memories. Yet the promise of her sense of humor, or the hope for it, drove all of us up to her room for hours every evening.

When her heart finally became too weak, when her asthma finally made her gasp for breath on every word, she was moved to the hospital. She died a week later, and none of us were surprised. But it was too soon, too sad for us all to handle rationally. So we turned into a caricature of the grieving British family, all shut doors and muffled crying. It didn't "do" to be sad, we didn't want the others to worry, we wanted to be strong for each other. Outwardly, we held hands and all told each other that we were "fine," that it was "her time," that she had been in pain and was now at peace. When my parents went to her funeral without me, I knew that they were trying to protect me.

From that moment on, I was watched a little more closely. My parents were worried that her death would be too much for me to handle, that it would break my spirit in some unforeseeable way. I was miserable and heartbroken, but I was more worried about my mum than about myself; I was more resilient than any of us expected. Yet my stutter was scrutinized more closely. When it didn't seem to be going away or getting any better, the connection was made. Death and stutter were tied together as if in some hideous three-legged race. We created our own explanation within the family. I stuttered as a result of my grandma's traumatic death, because of all the repressed emotion. It was no one's fault and everyone's fault.

So what did cause it? No one had any idea. Death was as good a stab in the dark as any. Twenty years later I finally put my grandma's ghost to rest and spent a year looking into the causes of stuttering, but when I was seven years old, we all just wanted it gone.

No one drew too much attention to it. My parents reacted as normally as they could. They smiled, waited, told me not to feel rushed. There were more hushed conversations than before, and everyone leaned in a little closer when I spoke, but otherwise very little notice was drawn to the fact that I periodically looked on the verge of an epileptic fit.

And that was how I believed I looked. I was no longer the normal child I had always been. I was strange. I made people nervous. Watching home videos of myself, I know that my stutter grew over time. I know that at seven years old I didn't have any of the curious behaviors that I would cultivate later in life. As time went by, I would try every possible trick to push through a word. If something worked once, I would employ it over and over again with the certainty of a religious convert. If I managed to expel a word one time after pinching my leg, I would do that faithfully until a bruise discouraged me. If a word came out after tracing the outline of each letter on the palm of my hand, I would assume that I had stumbled on a cure. If I swallowed before I spoke and my sentence followed fluidly, I would start swallowing manically until my mouth was drained of even a trace of saliva. Stamping my foot, flicking my head, squeezing my eyes shut. Anything to explode beyond the block and reach the other side. Everything worked once and then lost its power until I gave up in defeat.

But all of those secondary behaviors came later. At seven years old I hadn't yet developed any tricks to get around it. My reflexes told me to push, to jam the word out of my mouth, to follow my instincts. My breath gradually developed a raspy aspect, the desperate hoarseness of a committed smoker. The petrified observer would stare as my small mouth flew open, gaped, and then shuddered as the word hit a roadblock on the second letter. Reflexively a painful, scared expression would spread from my mouth to my eyes. I would glance down at the floor in embarrassment and then force myself to look up and lock eyes with my listener. As the words juddered, the chasm would widen and then—just as I worried that I might suffocate—it would pop out. I would gallop towards the rest of the sentence. Not quite finished, but not ready to continue. A halfhearted attempt to regain my dignity.

For most of the world the act of speaking is something barely considered; it is a subconscious event that happens as naturally as walking. However, whether or not we are aware of it, it is a tremendous event every time we decide to speak. Speaking is not a neatly localized event. It is not solely relegated to our lips or tongue or brain. Rather the process, from decision to execution, engulfs our whole bodies. When you cannot express yourself, speaking becomes a physically draining and emotionally traumatic struggle.

Imagine, for a moment, knowing what you want to say in your head, having the funniest joke at the ready or the most passionate argument. Then imagine going to speak and someone jamming a stopper into your throat. You get out a couple of words, and they do it again. And again. And again. Like some form of bizarre torture. Quickly enough you realize that it probably won't kill you, but your breathing is being tampered with and your body registers the affront on a life-threatening level. Stuttering throws off the whole respiratory system. In the words of speech therapist Phil Schneider, it messes with the "ballet of breathing." Stuttering occurs at the moment when there is a *lock,* a break in the continuity between speech and breathing. There is a loss of reciprocity. Both muscles decide to tighten at the same time and nothing moves. In essence, stuttering is a motor control glitch, but our reaction to it is far from simple. The glitch sets off a major fear response because our breathing system, our body's mechanism to keep us alive, is being attacked.

So the fear escalates and feeds the stutter. Stuttering is not a nervous impulse—experts no longer believe that emotional trauma causes stuttering—but it is certainly understood that it doesn't help matters along. Fear or passion act like lighter fuel on a smoldering fire.

As I began to stutter in every conversation, I gradually became afraid of speaking. I became nervous of what would happen when I opened my mouth, nervous of embarrassing myself or my parents. I started to ready myself for the feel of the strange clench in the middle of some unsuspecting word. Not only was I afraid, but I was also aware of the changing rhythm of my life. Once upon a time I would have asked for everything, jumped into any conversation, told anyone anything. Now that I stuttered I was more circumspect about throwing my voice around so wantonly.

Eating at the dinner table with family friends turned into an obstacle course. I began to weigh what I needed against what I wanted, deciding what was worth the effort and what was not. After one fateful evening, salt became a precious commodity, only asked for if the food was completely unpalatable. I had been perched on a cushion so that my head rose above the table. My parents had invited some friends over for a dinner party, the silver had been polished, the best glassware laid out, the tablecloth ironed the night before. Everyone had complimented my mum on the food, and my parents looked relaxed, safe in the knowledge that the night was a success. The conversation all around me had jumped from one person to the next, jokes spoken rapid-fire over my head, and three stories being told at once. In the safety of the background noise I had taken my chance. I tried asking the group once, very softly, and seeing if anyone heard. No one noticed, so I tugged on my dad's shirtsleeve and tried to ask him privately. I pulled him away from his conversation, "Ca ca ca ca ca ccc ca ca caan you p p p p p p p p pppp pa pa pa pa pa pa p p p . . ." Avid, as ever, to give me his full attention, he halted his conversation instantly. The one next to him stalled in the sudden quiet. Two lone people on the other side of the table were, mercifully, still engrossed in a story about an old friend, but everyone else was looking in my direction, watching me kindly and leaning towards me in anticipation.

I lost all taste for the stupid salt. I wished that I had never opened my mouth. Poised in expectation, I knew that they would all be disappointed by my paltry request. Salt did not deserve this kind of gravitas. It was meant to be a quick request, the sort that barely even broke the flow of conversation. I was tempted to give up, to wave it away. Instead, I barreled forward: "Ppp pass the sssssssss s s sss s sal sal sal salt?"

"Of course," everyone chimed in together.

They fought to reach for the shaker, five hands leant forward. The winning hand passed it towards me, as if I were being handed a prize. I accepted it gratefully. There was an awkward silence for a brief moment and then the conversations gradually resumed. I listened to the banter begin again, watched the beginning of some new story told by some dexterous tongue, and looked at the salt with disgust.

I doubt anyone else remembered those strange moments, those awkward times when my stutter shattered the rhythm of a conversation or left me dizzy and breathless. I wanted to forget, but they became etched in my memory, a depressing catalogue of everyday defeats. In their wake I gradually began to develop a new personality. As I left my old carefree persona behind, I began to learn what this new reality meant. Awareness hit me first, closely followed by abject fear, and then my lazy coping mechanisms finally arrived, a little late for the party.

Awareness was the strangest of all. It crept up on me and then lingered, this shadowy realization that something was different, but I couldn't say exactly what. When I went back to school after the incident with the ballet uniform, I was teetering on the edge of fear but not quite there. I was simply aware that something had changed, that I had no idea what would happen when I sat back down in the classroom.

I found out all too quickly. It was early May, the sun was streaming into the small school, and there was a lot of noise. Our small, polished shoes were tapping frantically on the floor as we tore off our coats in haste and ran into the classroom to tell each other all of the adventures of the past couple of weeks.

My uniform had been itchier that morning, I had been slower to get out of bed and quieter than normal on the car ride to school. But now that I was here, amid all my friends, I was fine. I could hear myself telling stories of my Easter holiday, running my words forward as I always had. Everything was normal. I was stumbling on a couple of letters, but it was nothing scary, and no one seemed to notice. I was on a roll, my earlier nerves gone, when the teacher clapped her hands together and asked everyone to take their seats.

She began to take the class register.

"Louisa-May?"

"Here."

"Soraya?"

"Here."

Suddenly *here* took on a life-threatening force. I couldn't say it. I knew I would fall apart on the *H*. I shifted in my seat. More "heres" mocked me and I knew my turn was approaching.

"Katherine?"

I knew that I had to come up with something. Two seconds had passed. She was looking up. I had to say something. "Yup!"

The teacher looked taken aback for a moment. "Yup?"

"Yup. I'm here." I knew that she hated the word *yup*, that it offended her delicate sensibilities, but I ignored the questioning, critical tone in her voice. I realized something else. I realized that I could say "Here" if I ran up to it and threw some other words in front.

The roll call ended and we all sat there in silence. She started to pace the room. She walked down the aisles between us and asked what we did during our Easter holiday. With her gait and occasional stare she started to take on the aspect of some menacing lioness on the hunt. I felt like prey, and I was scared that I had riled her with my cocky "Yup." I knew she would call on me. I felt sweat pool in the scratchy woolen armpits of my school uniform. I bit the eraser off the top of my pencil.

"Katherine? Could you tell us all one of your favorite pieces from your Easter holiday?"

Had I been able to summon the courage, I would have said "No," but that level of disobedience was not hardwired into me. Not yet anyway. I had been brought up to be polite and thoughtful, to remember my pleases and thank-yous, never to answer a teacher back. "Yup" was about as crazy as I got.

There was a part of me, the old cocky part of me, that still wanted to show off. To tell them everything—the good, the bad, and the ugly of my holiday. But I couldn't because the other part of me, the new stuttering part of me, now had hold of the reins. What would happen if I stuttered? What if I couldn't speak at all? How little could I get away with saying? By the time I opened my mouth to speak, my body was bloated with fear. "I went up t t t t t t t ttt t t t t t t t." My peripheral vision caught the girl next to me, caught her chair creak away from me in recoil. My ears heard the skirts fidgeting uneasily in their seats as they turned to look. I had an audience, everyone was facing me now. A couple of my friends were smiling, but most of them just looked a little confused, their eyebrows raised and their eyes darting towards the teacher for an explanation. I quickly decided that there was no way I was saying much more. I was conducting seven-year-old social suicide and I knew it. But I had to finish the sentence. The lioness would never let me get away with a half-finished attempt. I strangled myself free: "Ttt t t tto Scotland."

I was panting slightly now, beads of sweat were cresting down my forehead, but I was grateful that I had spit it out. An explosive sound from the girl next to me shattered my relief. She was sniggering, her lips wide and her head down. It was the same reaction that we all had when we watched someone trip or fall, the laughter directed at a fool.

My face grew red in reply. A blotchy red that smeared across my cheeks and reached up to my forehead. I froze in my seat and stared ahead. I couldn't smile, I couldn't pretend. I hadn't built up any walls to protect myself. I had been laughed at before and hadn't much minded. In fact, I had liked it. I had always laughed at others and myself. But this was different, because this time I didn't know what was funny. I wasn't in on the joke. This time I was the joke.

I hated it, but I had to do something. If they thought I was funny, then that was what I would be. I grabbed on to the notion and ran with it.

I heard the teacher ask me to carry on, to tell everyone more about Scotland. She spoke soothingly and slowly. I imagined that she was attempting to coax my tone out from wherever it had hidden. Her tone insulted me almost as much as the laughter, more perhaps. Giggling was better than pity. Anything was better than that.

I looked up at her. "Nn n n n nnot much." She looked down at me, waiting for more. I raised my palms to the ceiling and shrugged. The action made little sense, but it spoke loudly enough to tell her that I was refusing. The class sniggered at my cockiness. She waited; I stubbornly maintained my silence. Finally, she raised her eyebrows and turned to interrogate someone else. The class was once again filled with the chatter of voices: normal voices, high-pitched, excitable voices. I ripped a sticker off the front of my notepad.

As lonely and weird as I felt at the time, I now know that my experiences were not unusual. I have discovered that classrooms are popular backgrounds for stutterers to step into the light and cement themselves. Computer technician Bobby Childers's story is a telling one. It was only in the brutally honest confines of the classroom that other kids pointed out his stutter: "They said I talked funny." Kids have no social graces wired into them, they are judgment-free and entirely tactless. If they see something weird or funny, they will point and laugh. They won't carefully edge around the subject.

In the classroom you have an audience. You have to deal with a situation where everything is focused on your speech, on expressing yourself orally to your teachers and your peers. Away from the safety of home, where you can spend time running around or playing games with family, you have to start dealing with reactions that are not always pretty. The classroom is the first place that you begin to see what stuttering might mean for your life. The singer and songwriter Chris Trapper remembers waking up dreading school every day. "I used to always avoid class and skip school, especially if oral work came up. I would go to the nurse's office, anything not to confront the embarrassment and the humiliation," he remembers. "All the kids in school thought I was crazy. They thought I had some real problem, like I was retarded or something."

At school you are forced to realize that you are different. There's no escaping it. At a time in your life when all you want to do is fit in, you have to face the fact that everyone else is well aware of your strangeness. So you come up with a plan, a way to make it a little easier to carry on. At the time, I was ashamed of acting like the mute class clown, but it was the only exit route I could think of. And it seemed to work. Silently hilarious was a winning combination in my mind, just the cure I had been looking for. If I didn't speak, I didn't stutter. When I was silent, I was normal again.

CHAPTER 2

WHAT SHOULD WE DO?

London, June 1992

THE ICE CREAM shop is a rare treat. It is right next to the French Lycée in South Kensington, and everyone who works there acts like they are transported directly from Paris every morning. It is two minutes from my school and an afternoon visit feels thoroughly exotic on my walk home.

It is an unusually hot Wednesday afternoon in early June. The sidewalks are full of purple-uniformed children streaming out of the school and rushing home with their mums and nannies. I feel very special, as I have my two parents holding my hands. Fathers are a novel sight standing in the small school playground. I relish the occasion and swing my slightly too heavy body between them, wondering out loud how my dad has finished work so early today. He evades my question, "So what flavor ice cream are you going to have?"

The answer is obvious. Chocolate. It is always chocolate. But chocolate is difficult to say. As we walk in, I ask him to order chocolate for me. I watch him glance quickly at my mum and then back down to me, "That's okay, darling. You order it, you're a big girl now, so you get to order for yourself."

Normally, he is happy to order for me, and his answer throws me off. I contemplate ordering vanilla, which strikes me as disappointingly dull, or strawberry, which I think is truly disgusting. I refuse to squander my treat.

The line is two families deep. I watch as the children ahead of me are handed their glistening orbs in crisp sugar cones. I shuffle forward and push my sweaty fingers against the glass case as I look up at the young Frenchwoman.

"And what for you, mademoiselle?"

"The br br brown one."

She creases her brow and tilts her head sideways. "*Quoi?* Which one? This one?" She points at the coffee. I look up at her. Coffee? Granted, it is brown, but are the typical eight-year-olds that she serves really so sophisticated as to choose coffee over chocolate?

"No. This one." I point at the chocolate.

"Ze pistachio?"

This is not going well. I glance towards my parents. They shuffle uncomfortably but nod for me to carry on.

"No. This one." I point again.

"Ze praline?

Charades is clearly not my strong suit. "No, down one. Y Y yes, that one!"

"Ah, ze chocolat? Why did you not say so?"

I shrug. I have my reasons.

"And what kind of a cone would you like it in?"

When did they start offering a variety of cones? A normal cone, whatever kind of cone. Let's just get this over with.

"We have sugar cones, waffle cones, or you can have it in a cup."

I contemplate my options. Roll the sounds around silently in my head. Sugar and waffle sound delicious but impossible to say. I would love a cone. I can practically taste it crunching against the silky smoothness of the ice cream. I can picture myself savoring the chocolate at the bottom.

"Cup."

I watch in disgust as she starts scooping the ice cream. My mum leans forward and makes sure that I don't want a cone. She knows me too well. I shake my head. As always, my goal is to stutter as little as possible. I may not have exactly what I want, but I didn't stutter asking for it. I have no intention of sullying my success now.

As we walk out of the shop, I start to stick my spoon into my ice cream. It doesn't taste as good as normal. The plastic spoon ruins it. I would love to lick it out of the cup but that would just embarrass everyone. I play with it for a while and offer the resulting melted goop around. We walk down two blocks, and I toss it in a bin, half eaten. I want to rid myself of the evidence. I take both their hands in mine as we cross the street. The way they watch me does not escape my attention.

They have been asking me about my day, but I think I have successfully used the diversion of the ice cream to answer in a series of grunts and nods. It is probably the most I have said all day.

My self-taught strategy for combatting my stutter by not speaking might not be ideal, but it is the best I have come up with so far. I have taken to starring in my own silent movie. Unfortunately, mime is not my strong suit, and it only takes me so far. Conversations are a long-forgotten pastime. I have spent this day, like most others, sitting on the periphery, a little apart from the games around me. In the playground I took my apple slices to eat in the corner behind the big oak tree and watched people walk past the fence as my friends played tag out in the open. In class I had scribbled down the answers to the teacher's questions on my notepad but looked down furiously when she asked us to share our answers out loud. She had pushed me to share my thoughts. I had tried to resist, but she had forced me to speak, backed me into a corner. When I had opened my mouth, the syllables swelled in my throat. I had not been able to express even one complete word. I had said so little all day that the sound of the words shocked me as they crashed and fell in breathless spasms.

I can feel tears pricking my eyes as I remember how she frowned and looked at me pityingly. I wonder if perhaps she called my parents.

Despite a handful of dramatic failures, I think that I have managed to blend into the background pretty successfully over the past year. I play less with my friends and rush home at the end of the day. I have managed to reduce speaking to a functional necessity to get me through the day. I have succeeded in not stuttering as often, but my days are beginning to take on the melancholic aspect of someone far more world-weary. Having silenced myself, I'm becoming visibly depressed.

And yet, withdrawn as I have made myself, I am greedy for conversation, for any kind of connection. So I ask my parents short, open-ended questions as we walk. I fear that my strategy is obvious, but they consent to do the talking, for a while. As we walk past shops and restaurants, they regale me with stories from their daily adventures. I hear about lunches, meetings, car rides, and plans for the upcoming summer holidays. I nudge my dad and ask him what Donald Duck would think about the people he met this morning. He smiles, blows out his cheeks, and pushes his lips together as he launches into my favorite cartoon impersonation. I try to fulfill my role as Donald's translator, but soon enough I'm giggling too much to make any sense and Mum is laughing so hard that she starts crying.

As we swing onto our block I am feeling relaxed and confident again, so I pipe up, "W w w w w w www w w w w wwhat were you and Mum t t t t talking about tt th th the other night?" It is the longest sentence I have uttered for a while, but it has been on my mind all day. Quietly books on childhood development have started to push the Penguin Classics out of the way on our bookshelves. I have been noticing how conversations of "doctors" and "experts" are hushed around me as I walk into a room, replaced by sudden smiles. In a London town house of three, secrets are not the easiest thing to keep, and we normally shared everything. I have been imagining the worst.

They look at each other and we stop walking for a moment. The subject is bigger than I have imagined. I start to shift from foot to foot on the pavement and wonder how long it would take me to run home. "We just want to chat to you about speech therapy, darling." My mum looks unsure, readying herself for an argument.

The two words were worse than I had thought. My dad sinks down onto his haunches so he can look me in the eye, "The doctor says that eighty percent of kids grow out of this, but you haven't and we want you to try out this new therapy. It's at the Michael Palin Centre in London, and it is only two weeks out of the summer holiday." My brain has frozen and the only word that cuts through my stalled psyche is the name Michael Palin. My dad watches the name register and I hear him tell me that the actor has given his name to the program, that stuttering is a cause close to his heart. My hearing is muffled by the clattering fear in my brain, but I hear him joke that we may get the chance to meet the Monty Python actor someday. My mum joins in from my other side, "It will be all kids, and you can just see how it goes."

They say it all so calmly. I can see how much they want to help, and yet all I hear is that I have "failed" at growing out of something, that it is obvious to everyone that I am weird and that I need to be fixed. I feel ashamed.

I quickly find out how anger affects my speech. I tell them that I don't want to go. They tell me that they have my best interests at heart, that it would be best if I gave it a shot. Then I begin to shout. I don't care what the neighbors think as curtains twitch from nearby windows. I don't stutter once.

Screaming, focused anger makes for a great bedfellow with fluency. So I scream and cry and release all the pent-up anger and embarrassment that have been held captive in my small body for the past year. I have argued with my mum before, but I have never shouted at my dad. I can see that I am hurting them both. I storm back to the house, wait for them to open the door, and then, attempting to regain my fierce independence, march up to my room.

I begin to pack. I grab my Paddington Bear suitcase and throw in my favorite threadbare T-shirt. I have told my parents that I would rather leave the house than go to speech therapy. I have offered them an ultimatum, but they haven't backed down quite how I was hoping. Unwilling to lose face, I am now contemplating my potential new life on the streets. My mum pokes her head tentatively round the door. "Would you like me to help you pack?"

"I don't need your help. I'll be fine on my own."

She nods sagely and walks in anyway. She holds up my underwear. "You may want a few pairs of these."

I agree. This will be tougher than I thought.

"You may want a few trousers and skirts, too."

I may have been angry, but she did have a point. I throw in the extra clothes and a favorite pair of boots. I have never packed before, and it is harder than I imagined.

"Would you like me to make some sandwiches for you? You might get hungry, darling."

I nod and she walks slowly out the door. I can feel some tears welling up. This is not going quite as expected. Mum is a tougher negotiator than I had bargained for. Neither of us is backing down, and the thought of leaving the house is becoming markedly less tempting by the moment. My suitcase is already rather heavy, and I have left almost everything behind.

I start to pull it down the stairs. It jogs and jerks forward, pulling me down ungracefully behind it. My mum is waiting in the sitting room holding my favorite teddy. I can't believe I left him behind. She holds him out, "I thought you might want Brown Bear to keep you company."

I look at her holding the teddy out towards me and realize that I don't have much of a plan of what I will do once I step outside. My resolve shifts and then falls apart. "Mama. I'm sorry. I don't want to leave."

"Darling, I don't want you to go either. I'd miss you terribly." I sense that she knew I would never leave, but I can see that her eyes are glistening with the threat of tears.

She leans down and hugs me, and I smell the familiar smell of her. I hold back for a moment and then reach my stubby arms around her. She holds me out so I can see her face. "But, darling, we really want you to try out this speech therapy course. Your stammer, I mean your speech, it just . . ." She takes a breath, starts again. "Your dad and I want to help you and this place is the best. Will you give it a try? For us. You never know: it might be fun."

She has taken it too far at the end. I doubt very much that it will be fun. But I relent. I'll go. She helps me drag my suitcase back up the stairs.

The worst thing is that I am fully aware what the word *therapy* means. It means that I am abnormal. It means that I need help. It implies a level of madness, something uncontrollable that needs to be tamed. In my mind it is an accusation, something to be kept secret. I assume that if any of my friends find out that I am going to speech therapy, they will immediately place me further down the lower orders of the school hierarchy. I will be pityingly lumped together with the fat kid, the kid who speaks to herself, and the one who smells like she has not yet been introduced to a shower.

So "therapy" is something to be kept secret. To be kept at a distance. To be kept away from words like *stammer* or *stutter*. I quickly learn that the words are interchangeable, that there is no difference between them, that both of them hold the dangerous power of taboo. They are swearwords whispered at me, although rarely, from the sides of the playground as I walk by. But at home they are never given air time. Even now, even as we talk about therapy, the stutter, or stammer, is barely spoken of.

And yet, although I am angry and deflated by the thought of going to speech therapy, I'm glad. I'm glad that someone has brought my stutter out and pushed it into the limelight. Deep down I am glad that someone has acknowledged that something is happening, that it has a name, that it might have a treatment. Because the silence is the most oppressive thing of all. Not only my own silence, the lonely, frustrating sense that the world is moving past me, but also the silence of everyone around me. I am strangling myself to talk and muting myself and fighting through conversations, and no one is saying anything about it.

• • •

THERE IS no handbook for what to do when your child starts stuttering. As a parent, you assume that you should know how to fix things. And if you can't fix something, you feel guilty. You feel like you must have done something wrong, that you have somehow failed as a parent.

Stuttering is a messy and complicated condition. Sometimes it is even difficult to diagnose. Much of the time it does not sound like the simple syllable repetition that we have come to expect. The cartoonish sounds that we are taught to associate with stuttering are relatively rare in real life. Stuttering can look like an internal struggle. It can look forgetful or like some kind of perpetual spasm. It can happen on every word, or it can be hidden in certain situations and raise its head only forcefully and sporadically.

Some parents can't tell that there is even a "real" problem. Others know that there is something wrong, but they cannot get the clinical world to acknowledge their concerns, let alone to treat their child. Electrical engineer Nick Richard remembers the first time his mum took him to see a speech pathologist, "She had me describe a bunch of pictures. I knew that she was trying to get me to stutter, but it was such easy stuff that I didn't. She said, 'He's fine.' Next my mum took me to a local hospital for a number of months, and there they did hearing tests and speaking tests, and I never stuttered once. They said we can't help you at all. The tests were always so basic that there was no real reason to stutter. So I was never diagnosed as a stutterer until I was thirteen. That was the first time I stuttered in front of a speech therapist."

Every parent is given different advice from their pediatricians and speech therapists, and every parent handles his or her child's stutter in their own way. Some people, my parents included, were advised not to let on that they were concerned. Their doctor told them to smile at me, to look me in the eye, to always look interested, to let me finish my words. They were advised not to frown, not to make me feel like I was doing anything wrong, not to repeat my sentences back to me. The idea was that if none of us drew attention to it, then the stutter would simply cease to exist.

Naturally, they were protective; they rescued me whenever they could. They spoke for me when I asked them to, they answered the telephone, they did all they could to create a world within a world where I was free from feeling bad about myself. They were doing the right thing, the best they could.

I was lucky. I know of some parents who shouted at their children, who told them to spit out their words, who cut them off and looked away when they started speaking. Some gave in to their frustrations and snapped, telling their children to stop stuttering, as if they had a choice in the matter. As ludicrously Dickensian as it sounds, I know of kids who were punished for stuttering, children who were hit for not speaking "right" and told off for putting on the stutter to get attention. Jamie Rocchio remembers her parents telling her everything from "Go to your room if you can't talk right" to "I'm not going to listen to you if you stutter" and "If you can't say it, don't talk." The singer Bill Withers expresses that same sentiment in much more understated terms, telling me that he "didn't grow up with a whole lot of 'you can' people around."

Some parents are told to give their children pills. To medicate the stutter out of them. Some kids are prescribed relaxants for years of their adolescence. From the age of nine, lifeguard and martial arts expert Matt Murray remembers being "on antidepressants for eight years." My doctor was a little more old-school than Matt's. From his stately, antique-filled London practice, he told my parents to wait and see. He reassured them that I would grow out of "it," that "it" would go away on its own. My stutter was just another milestone on the road of childhood development. A temporary thing. He had statistics on his side. Three out of four kids would prove him right.

However, I was not growing out of it. More important, I was losing confidence at an alarming rate. Every day I was sliding further into myself and moving further away from my previously carefree personality. Every day my speech was drifting further away from the fluent voice in my head. It was a protection thing: I needed to become introverted to face the difficulty of my new reality. In much the same way the naturally extroverted filmmaker Daniel Kremer remembers, "I was very withdrawn, I was well removed from most social activities. I didn't want to talk for fear of embarrassment. It used to take me two minutes to say my name."

The transformation was not pretty. My mum and dad couldn't just sit around and do nothing. They were watching their child, who had once been bubbly and rambunctious, become quieter by the day. So outwardly they acted like everything was normal, but inwardly they worried. I may have been anxious about my new speech, but so were they, perhaps more so. When I was eight years old, my mum started to telescope my future. What would my life be like? Would I always make friends? Would I be bullied? What kind of a job would I have? While I was playing with my impressive collection of My Little Ponies, Mum was worrying about whether I would find a good chap to marry.

So they called around, they did their research, and they found the best speech therapy they could. And they signed me up because it seemed like the right thing to do, the right medicine, the right doctor to see. None of us had any idea. I didn't know why I stuttered, and we didn't have any precedents. There were no family members that we knew of, no one to learn from, no friends to call up. So speech therapy was a way for them to help me, a way to feel a little less helpless.

THE METAL hits the back of my knees and sticks awkwardly to my thighs. My skirt is too short, and the chair feels cold and clinical against my bare legs. I pull down on my hem and look around at the circle of preadolescent boys in front of me. I am the only girl in the room. For the first time, I am aware that I am a minority within a minority, that stuttering girls are rare, that the condition latches on to men far more commonly.

I look at the boy directly ahead of me. He looks as scared as I feel. His forehead is shining in the light of the fluorescent bulbs as the boy next to him pushes and struggles against the weight of his name. My eyes glance across and, in the torturous silence of the large room, the speech therapist looks directly at him.

She is about the same age as my mum. An adult, but not a really old one. She has pretty brown hair and kind eyes. I like her. I like the way she smiles at everyone. I like that she told us that stuttering wasn't our fault, that we might sometimes have some difficulty speaking but that there are options to make it easier. She has neatly labeled our stutters, defining the breathless pauses as "blocks" and the bubbling words as "repetitions." She has told us that she is going to teach us a few techniques to smooth out our voices. I was hopeful when she was talking to us this morning, but now that we have started practicing the techniques, I am less certain.

"Try again, John. Remember to use the easy onset we spoke about. This time try to almost whisper the first letter and then hold it as you elongate and slide into the next letters. 'Jooooooooooohn.'" The way she says it, "John" sounds suspiciously more like "on." He is visibly drained but looks across at her hopefully. I cross my fingers under my chair, wishing that her languid, fluent speech would somehow enter his voice. He stutters on the *J* and then stops. He starts again and this time he merges his name into one long exhaled breath. With his ordeal over he leans back in his seat and looks challengingly to his left. If he has to go through it, he is damn sure that no one else is going to find it easy. The boy in front of me looks like he is considering running, but we all know that there's nowhere to go. We all know that we are stuck in the clinical room of this North London institution until our parents come to save us at the end of the day. With a resigned look on his face, and the sound of the speech therapist's soothing voice wafting towards him, he begins. It comes out more easily for him. He lays his words out across the air, talking to her with the rhythm and speed of a barfly.

We sound ridiculous. If we have to talk like this to be accepted in the outside world, I'd rather be silent. Bucking the status quo, the next boy refuses to use the technique, and it makes me look up. I watch transfixed as he struggles through his name. It is like holding up a mirror and looking on as my own facial contortions and scratched CD–style of speech are viciously played back to me. I force my eyes away and hear the speech teacher calmly asking him to use the technique. He does so, and bitterly I think that he sounds only a little better.

My turn comes next. My girly whisper stands out amongst the room of preadolescent male voices. "Kkkkkkkkkkkkaaaaa aaatttttherine." I give her what she wants. I don't like the way I sound, I find it immensely more exhausting than stuttering, and I can't imagine ever using this way of talking in my life outside of the room. But I don't want to fail. I want her to like me and I want her to tell my parents how well I am succeeding. I know that I am just playing the game, just going through the motions of changing my speech patterns. I hear her melodic voice share some well-meant praise with the room and squirm in my chair.

Every day of the course I become angrier. The treatment is not as easy as I was hoping, and I am not seeing any difference. It just makes me feel weird. I feel like I'm missing out on my summer holiday, like I'm being punished. During the days

I play the part of the doting student, and at night I vent my rage by screaming at my mum. I watch her face fall and later go to sleep with that image burning a hole in my dreams. I am a midget-sized version of Jekyll and Hyde.

The truth is that I don't want to be a part of the freak show. That is how I see it. At eight years old I don't want to be associated with other stutterers. I don't want to join their motley crew.

My childhood experience is not all that unusual. I have met others who balked as their parents signed them up for group therapy, who hung their heads in shame as they were taken from class to see the school speech therapist, who refused to talk to any other stutterers they came across. You have to be ready for speech therapy, ready for change. If you're not, then the whole experience feels like an affront, an imposition on your body.

In the therapy room, I start to get competitive. I watch as the boys start to improve, as they start to break free. In truth, we are all improving in the strange confines of the therapy course. It is easy to improve in the safety of those four walls: like inmates we're all becoming institutionalized. I begin to like them, begin to enjoy sharing stories, and I start to picture us playing together after school. As the end of the course approaches, that moment we have all longed for, we start to dread going back out into the real world.

Statistics will later break us into two groups. Those who "recover" and those who don't. For those children who recover, either the therapy is successful or their hormone-filled bodies naturally engulf their stutter and replace it with

a caramel-smooth voice. As they grow up, their stutter is reduced to a hazy memory tucked away in some dusty crevice.
Years later it will still be there in the shadows, but they will
rarely think about it, and it will rarely rear its head to make
an appearance.

At the time I think I am one of the chosen few. As furi-
ous as I am, as much as I tell everyone that I don't need to be
fixed, I can't help but notice that my speech has changed. I'm
not just fluent every now and then. Not just fluent when I use
the speaking techniques. No, I am completely and utterly fluent. The realization makes me giddy. I have graduated into the
world of people again, and I am free to ask for anything. My
parents can't shut me up.

As the days pass, my parents remind me to practice the techniques. In demonstration they pause, they talk more slowly,
they do all the things they were told to do to support me. They
gently tell me that I should go back to a refresher course in a
couple of months. I stubbornly refuse. I tell them that there is
no chance that I will ever put a foot back in that room.

I am triumphantly fluent and adamant that my stutter is
gone for good. Whatever misgivings my parents may harbor,
they can't hide their own jubilation. A smile breaks across
their faces every time I call up my grandparents or invite a
friend over for supper. As usual, our house is full of family friends, and every person I speak to marvels at my new
speech. I am an everyday miracle, and I revel in the attention.
But I'm doomed for a fall. It comes more quickly than anyone
could have predicted.

Two weeks after the course, I start to taste the familiar shape of the stuttered words billowing forward in my mouth. Deep in my brain, behind the novel self-confidence, I have always doubted the technique. My stutter is more powerful than a few weeks with a kind speech therapist. It is stronger than she is, as stubborn as I am. I may not be shocked, but disappointment racks my body. I bitterly watch the confused faces of everyone who has been fooled by my attack of fluency. I hear my parents' questions. Why am I not still using the technique? Why is it not working anymore? I don't have any answers. We all assume that the technique is foolproof. After three weeks at the intensive speech therapy course, the technique is beyond reproach and, if the technique is not at fault, then all eyes turn to me. Do I not want it badly enough? Am I not determined enough to make it work?

Failure becomes a new word in my vocabulary. I held fluency for a moment, but it slipped through my fingers. I let it fall out of my grasp. Stuttering is no longer something that just happened to me. It is now something that I have tried to overcome and botched. My sense of self has been altered. I am an underachiever, a loser, and a disappointment. For all of us, fluency has been the goal, and every stuttered word that spills forth makes me feel more guilty, more like a failure. I shout at my parents when they remind me to use my technique, I run up to my room to escape their concern. I hide behind forts that I build out of pillows and duvets, and I rebuild the walls that I had created around my stutter. I refuse to talk about it, refuse to let anyone else broach the subject. I can handle my own guilt, but I am ill-prepared to carry everyone else's disappointment.

Bitterly I hate the course. I vehemently believe that it has cruelly tricked us all. It has forced us all to see that stuttering is my own fault, and it has made us picture what life would be like if I were normal.

CHAPTER 3

MOLDED BY MIRRORS

I WATCH MY MUM absently push a stray strand of hair behind her ear. She throws her head back at a joke I can't hear, and her laughter bubbles to the sides of our living room. The group around her bend their foreheads towards her conspiratorially. A couple of women in the room lean backwards to catch a glimpse, to see who's having all the fun, who they should make their way towards. She is holding a tray of appetizers, and I watch her gracefully make her exit and begin to squeeze between the groups of twos and threes.

She puts down her tray as she leans over to hug a new couple that have walked in the front door. I see a glimpse of the teeming rain outside before they push the door shut. I watch her take their coats and drape them over her arm as she introduces the pair to a woman who, moments ago, was wandering around aimlessly. She looks grateful, relieved to have a conversation to ground her. As Mum moves to leave the conversation, to find a resting place for the drenched woolen coats, a hand touches her arm, and she glances over her shoulder. Her shifting ankles spin her heels slightly, a drink slips from the hand of someone behind and splashes red wine towards her. The flying liquid leaves a dark stain down the back of her blue dress. Friends cluck around her, and the culprit looks crestfallen, but Mum waves the incident off lightheartedly.

I watch my dad lean across to take the coats, I hear him boom a welcome to some new guest and turn around to retrieve the thread of some past conversation. I see him point up towards the Yemeni sword that hangs incongruously in our sitting room. I imagine him telling the story I've heard so many times before, the tale of how my parents met, of him working as a banker in Sanaa, of my mum coming to Yemen on holiday, of love at first sight. I strain my ears to catch my favorite piece of the story, the years of love letters, but my hearing isn't up to the task and I try to see where Mum has gone instead. I catch her slipping between the groups, and I hope that she will come over to me, that she'll sneak upstairs with me so I can help her rub out the stain. I see an old friend arrive, arms outstretched, and I know that the blemish on her dress is forgotten for now.

I have been looking forward to the party for weeks. In the part of me that makes me my mother's daughter, I am drawn to the boisterous, joyful feeling of a crowd. I love the frenzied excitement of the last few minutes before the first guest arrives. Even as a child, I can taste the enticing potential for who, or what, the night might hold. And yet, I am my father's daughter too, proud of the legendary parties that we host but more inclined to gravitate towards small groups of old friends and family.

I had slipped away to the bathroom and am lingering on the stairs when my mum sees me. I wave and she waves back. I'm still thinking whether or not I want to rejoin the fray, whether I want to relinquish the safety of my vantage point.

We wink at each other, and she mouths something I can't quite understand. As she starts walking towards me, another conversation pulls her in, and she rolls her eyes secretly. Her signal that she is on her way, that she'll make it soon, that her job as host is never done. But we both know that she is in her element here. My mum is the most social person I know, the easiest person in the world to talk to.

I see her point at someone across the room coming towards me. A warning gesture. A watch out, ready yourself. I turn my head in time to see one of my dad's business friends walking towards me. She looks like she's on a mission. I assume she is someone's wife. Unsuccessfully, I try to remember her name.

"Katherine." She pulls me in for an awkward hug. "How are you?"

I opt for a safe. "Great, thanks. And you?"

"Good." I stare at the complex pattern of her heavy tartan shirt as she starts to tell me about her husband, about their recent holiday to Italy. I half listen. I look up and catch my mum's eye again, and she looks at me questioning. I smile back. I want her to think I'm okay, that I'm as socially dexterous as she is. As much as I would love to have her by my side,

I want her to think that I can handle it on my own. I watch her nod and smile as she slips through the crowd, downstairs towards the kitchen. The woman touches my arm to secure my attention again, "I hear that you went on a speech therapy course. How was it?"

"Fine. Thank you."

"You know, I have a nephew who stuttered. He went to this great therapy, and now he's cured. Amazing, isn't it. Apparently, it is just about learning how to breathe properly."

I begin to nod. Simple. Just breathe properly. What the hell am I doing? Why can't I do that?

"So how is your speech these days?"

"Good. Tha Tha . . ."

"Relax, Katherine. Take a deep breath." She takes her deep breath herself. Just in case I don't understand her complicated instructions. A little show-and-tell exercise.

"My speech is g g g g g . . ."

She carries on deep breathing for a while and then decides to jump in. "Good?"

"Yes. It's good."

She doesn't need to say anything. Her face speaks for her. Her eyes grow wide, she frowns and then half smiles knowingly. She pities my delusion. Good? Really? Certainly not great. Not cured like her nephew.

"Are you practicing your techniques? Are you practicing them every evening and every morning? I know that my nephew had to practice a lot."

"I am. I practice e e e e e e . . ."

"Every day?"

Does this woman finish everyone's sentences? If she does, I might forgive her. I wonder if her nephew appreciates it when she says his words. Unfortunately, her guess was wrong. I wasn't going to say "every day." Every day wasn't true. I was going to say "every now and again." But she had said "every day," not me. And I didn't want to run up at the word again.

"Yup."

For a moment I feel relieved. Inadvertently she has saved me. And then I feel pathetic, as if my words are not worth waiting for. I am annoyed that she has stolen my language, that she hasn't taken the time to listen, to wait for a couple of extra seconds. Now I am caught in the lie.

"You practice every single day?"

What is this, an inquisition?

"Yup."

She pauses for a moment. I try to think of something to say to change the subject. I try to imagine what my parents would say. My mind is disappointingly blank. I decide the best thing to do is to launch into a very British discussion about the weather, but she beats me to it.

"Have you ever thought about hypnosis?"

As I shake my head, she starts to speak, almost to herself, "I know a good hypnotist, I should mention it to your mum. She's had lots of success with trauma victims. Regression therapy and all that."

Then she seems to remember something.

"Before the therapy fixed him, my nephew used to tell me that he didn't stutter at all when he sang."

I'm starting to hate her nephew.

"Have you ever tried singing your words? I know a great singing tutor that I could introduce you to."

I can feel my toes clench in my patent leather shoes. I pull down on the hem of my dress. What does she expect me to say to that? I shake my head, "Thanks for the ad ad advice. I have to go help my mum in the kitchen." I walk away before she launches into a show tune and pulls me in for an impromptu duet.

"STUTTER IS a cage made of mirrors," writes the poet Phil Kaye. "Every 'Are you ok?,' every 'What you say,' every 'Come on kid, spit it out,' is a glaring reflection you cannot escape."

When we are young we are molded by the reactions of others. As the singer Bill Withers explains, "The first learning we all go through is learning how to manage other people's reactions and other people's perceptions." We see our faults and our successes in their eyes, in their posture. As I rounded out my adolescence and looked forward to becoming a teenager, I was well aware that stuttering was a very public problem. It exposed itself every time I opened my mouth; it laid me bare to be judged.

"My stutter stopped when I went blind," remembers the novelist and nature writer Ted Hoagland. Sitting in the fading light of his Vermont cabin, he explains, "I couldn't see people's faces so I either had to stop stuttering or shut down and die in a social sense." Ted's voice may have been loosened out of necessity, but I wonder how much of his voice was freed because he no longer saw the reactions of others. Very few people stutter when they are standing alone in a room speaking to themselves, so how much did Ted's blindness free him from reacting to the perceptions of others?

We all know pity when we see it. We know attraction and repulsion and anger. Our sensitivity to others is instinctual, woven deep into our survival psyche. At a young age, we constantly search for approval, for validation that we are doing the right thing, that we are growing in the "right" way. We are testing to see what makes people laugh or cry or give praise. With stuttering we quickly learn that no reaction is best. We gravitate towards those who can see beyond the mask of stuttering. Those who wait patiently, who tell us jokes, who show no trace of discomfort, those who listen to us the way they listen to everyone else.

But there are always those who can't control their expressions or who choose not to. Those whose faces crease into a frown, who draw back their eyelids in shock.

Flawed as we are, it is those reactions that tend to stick with us. The teacher who determinedly looks away from us and stares at her chalkboard whenever we speak, the waiter who awkwardly stares down at the floorboards, or the receptionist who taps her fingers impatiently and looks around the room for someone to rescue her. They are the ones who make us feel too monstrous to behold.

If someone looked at me pityingly once, or snapped, or smirked, I was always on the lookout for a repeat performance. Like many people who stutter, I became hyperaware of the perceptions of others. I became afraid of what I would see. I started to read every reaction at the level of an expert mind reader.

"Stuttering forces you to be self-conscious and to think about how other people are perceiving you," explains film director Jeff Blitz. "That can be a really uncomfortable thing to be confronted with, but it can also be helpful. Stutterers can be very sensitive to people's unspoken perceptions. You get used to reading body language. When someone looks a certain way, even if it is fleeting and subtle, we tend to lock on to that kind of thing quickly."

I wonder what people think of when they picture a "stutterer." Do they picture someone a little shy and nervous? Do they feel sorry for someone afflicted with a stutter? Do they worry that it is contagious? Do they not want to be associated with someone who stutters? Perhaps I'm being rude. Perhaps no one thinks any such things. For most of my life I knew what everyone was thinking, or I thought I did. I worried that they assumed the mottled and maimed pace of my speech represented my entirety. I worried that they thought that all stutterers were alike, that we were all something to be pitied and shied away from.

When I was growing up, I had shop clerks walk away from me awkwardly. I had call center operators tell me to repeat myself until I was screaming hoarsely down the line. I had waiters tell me to "spit it out" and elderly relatives ask me to "calm down" or "speak slower," as if stuttering were so easily controlled, as if my speech was caused by petty foolishness. Computer programmer Gianni Jacklone bitterly remembers the annoyance he felt when people reacted to his stutter by saying, "I thought you were fucking with me." As if stuttering were a joke, something put on to make people laugh and draw attention to yourself. As if we were all just playing the role of a stutterer for fun.

I always wondered if those same people would have asked a blind person to "focus in" or recommend that a deaf person "listen a little harder." Unfortunately, stuttering is not always seen as a "valid" condition, whatever that may mean. All too often it is judged and seen as a personal weakness, a character flaw rather than a disability. Stutterers may be seen as unintelligent, as limited, as inadequate in some way. Stuttering is not generally linked up with the most attractive of attributes. It is unusual but not quite unusual enough. In most adults, the delivery of their speech betrays who they are or what they are feeling. So, in people's minds, stuttering may look like something they have seen before, something they recognize in their own stumbled speech.

It might appear unintelligent, indicative in some way of stupidity or mental weakness. "I was held back in fourth grade because of my stammer," remembers Marc Shell. Today Marc is a writer, literary critic, and the Irving Babbitt Professor of Comparative Literature and a professor of English at Harvard University. However, growing up in Montreal in the late 1950s and early '60s, "the school board believed stuttering to be a certain sign that I was stupid." Michael Palin remembers angrily believing as a kid that his Cambridge-educated dad was always passed over for promotion because of his stutter. In his opinion, "the biggest misconception is that stutterers are slow, that they speak slowly so they are slow."

It might appear shifty and nervous. When someone is shy or anxious, they tend to mumble, to trip over their words incoherently. When someone is not being entirely honest, they tend to look down or their voice breaks and they repeat themselves. There is an assumption that, if you're telling the truth, if you are confident, your voice will flow smoothly. Gerard Enright, a retired NYC Teamster, remembers describing a car accident and the policeman interrupting, "You can't trust him. He can't even speak; he's lying."

It might appear angry and unstable. When someone stomps their foot or spasms to push out a word, it can look violent and desperate and, in some cases, their personal frustration can be sadly misconstrued. "Back in Nigeria there was an accepted belief that people who stuttered were short-tempered or had a short fuse," remembers the distinguished Nigerian pediatrician Philip Ozuah. "It was widely accepted that they would lash out at you when they got angry because they couldn't express themselves verbally."

Worst of all, it might seem like nothing at all. A well-meaning listener might brush it off as nothing, or tell you that they stutter, too, that they mess up their words when they're nervous or overexcited. It is kind, in a way; it is their way of lumping us all together, of bringing us into the group. And yet it belittles the problem, it assumes that we are senselessly making a big deal out of something minor. The truth is that stuttering is a real problem with real casualties. The Dominic Barker Trust, set up to fund research and support for stuttering, is a reminder of how horrifyingly real stuttering can be. In 1994, at the age of twenty-six, Dominic walked outside with a shotgun and killed himself. He had two university degrees in agriculture and economics, but he believed that people didn't see his ability. He believed that he was marred by his stutter, that his accomplishments were always overshadowed by the intrusion of it. In 1997, his parents set up the charity in his memory.

Many times the most damning misconceptions are the ones we assume others have of us or the ones we have of ourselves. "I used to think I had a demon in me," remembers the Mexican teacher Mele Rael. Sitting in his quiet home in Arroyo Hondo, New Mexico, he told me, "People say that if they cut the muscle on the bottom of your tongue that you can speak. You don't want to know how many times I held scissors there." I've heard of people who pressed the handles together, who were desperate enough to try anything, however barbaric, to free themselves of the stutter.

So often, particularly when we are growing up, we are in the dark together with our listeners. When I was much younger, I had no idea how to present myself, and my audience had no idea how to react. Unfairly I battled their best attempts. I broke pens, replied with a saccharine smile, silenced any mention of my stutter, and tried to explain myself if the conversation was forced upon me. As I grew older, my reactions ran the gamut from the polite to the profane. As difficult as I found their words and their troubled expressions, as much as I tallied the depressing list of misconceptions that my audience seemed to harbor, there was only one reaction that I was truly afraid of. Only one that I had no script for.

I didn't much like the idea of someone walking away from me, but I was terrified of mockery. I was always afraid that stuttering was funny, that this thing I had been born with had turned me into a comedian. On the rare occasion that I heard giggles or the sound of my stumbled words mimicked back to me, I was devastated. I felt criticized and demeaned. In the words of author Benson Bobrick, "my heart hardened" against my tormentor. Those were moments when I saw, inescapably, that I was laughable.

There were times when it was malicious, but more often than not, I can see now that it was born of embarrassment, of nervousness and shock. As speech therapist Phil Schneider puts it, "Laughter is usually not criticism. It is usually discomfort or surprise." Stuttering is strange and uncomfortable, so people laugh to ease their own discomfort. If we are honest, many disabilities can be seen in that light, and yet stuttering is one of the few that is openly mocked. Why?

It may be too simple to blame the media, but Hollywood remains the harbinger of taste for many, and the film industry has done precious little to correct these misconceptions. Hollywood has long pegged disfiguration to villainous characters, and stuttering has been used as a visual cue to symbolize everything from insanity and abuse (*One Flew Over the Cuckoo's Nest*) to personal weakness, ineptitude, and violent moral corruption (*Primal Fear*). Even in the recent Oscar-winning film *The King's Speech,* the script writers leant heavily on a variety of outdated and tired stereotypes. In the therapist's office, viewers are encouraged to believe that the king's stutter came from a variety of incidents in his childhood; his use of corrective splints on his legs; being forced to overcome his left-handedness; undergoing virtual starvation at the hands of a spitefully cruel nanny; facing the mockery of his older brother; reacting to the sustained verbal abuse from his father.

The film may reinforce a variety of misconceptions, and yet its merits outweigh its flaws. It is bolstered by Colin Firth's gritty determination and dignity in the midst of a gulping stutter and Geoffrey Rush's contextual evocation of a therapist's humanity and compassion. More important, it shows us how the difficulty of speaking with a stutter makes the king stand apart, how his hard-won public voice can command a nation. Before films such as *Rocket Science* and *The King's Speech*, filmmakers largely reinforced their own take on stuttering as a personality disorder and lazily used it for a cheap laugh.

I remember the first time I saw what a joke my condition was, what a joke I was. I was about to watch a movie that my mum had told me not to see—*A Fish Called Wanda*. The name was intriguing, I had no idea what it meant.

I remember giggling nervously on the sofa with my friends as someone pressed Play. I can still feel how we pinched each other and fidgeted as the opening credits showed the London scenes.

I was woefully unprepared. My stomach turned as Michael Palin said his first line, "Hello, W W W W W W W Wanda." His next line was worse. Not just a stumble over words but some head throwing, mouth clenching, and eye shutting thrown in for effect. His character, Ken, had a severe stutter. Michael was acting it too well, making it too real.

Before I could rearrange my features into a calm repose Kevin Kline's character burst onto the screen. It was immediately clear that Otto's role was that of the stutterer's worst enemy, the malicious and sadistic tormentor. Laughing, he verbalized what we were all thinking; he turned it into a swearword, "Well, that's quite a stutter you've got there, Ken." Then he became damningly condescending: "It's okay, it doesn't bother me."

The opening scenes set the stage for the next ninety minutes. Every stuttering stereotype was played out in Technicolor. Ken the stutterer was awkward, nervous, and reclusive. Otto was the malicious bully. The two other characters took on the sympathetic and indifferent listeners respectively. All the perceptions I had of myself, all the perceptions I assumed others had of me, were confirmed as I watched a microcosm of my life unfold.

I sat trapped, rigidly staring at the flickering screen. I felt the burning heat of shame travel from my neck to my cheeks. The minutes crept across the face of the clock above the telly. I dared not look away. I dared not see the poorly hidden glances from my friends. I dared not let on how much the film was breaking me. I laughed as loud as I could to fill up the silence.

At the time all I could think was, Why? Why had Michael done it? He seemed like such a nice chap. What had stutterers ever done to him? Many years later, I found out.

Having agreed to an interview, I was sitting in his central London office as he told me how his father stuttered, how he had grown up in the shadow of his father's speech. He told me that he took on the role of Ken because he believed that he was best placed to play him, because he knew the condition more intimately than most. And yet he had questioned himself, he had questioned if he was doing the right thing. "I don't think I would have done it if my father had still been alive. I think it might have been quite hurtful," he said. "I think if he had seen it, he would have felt like I was rubbing it in and making a joke about him personally."

He finally decided to take on the role because he believed "that the real problem was that no one acknowledged stammering. By not talking about it, it made stammerers seem like people from another planet with some strange condition that made them a victim. So it was important to bring a stammer into a mainstream character in a movie and make him a real, rounded, three-dimensional person rather than just a talking joke. At the end of the film Ken wasn't one of these awful people, but he wasn't a saint either."

Years later I could understand his rationale. I could appreciate how worthwhile it was to put a character who stuttered in the limelight, to open the conversation. However, at the age of ten, all I saw was his painfully accurate portrayal of a stutterer. I didn't see Ken as a three-dimensional character, I didn't stick around to see the end, to watch him crush his tormentor with a steamroller and bury him in wet cement. I might have liked the movie more if I had.

Instead, I was already out the door, already promising myself that I would never speak of the movie to anyone. I had already called my dad, was already waiting for him to come and pick me up. To save me.

CHAPTER 4

TACTICAL WARFARE

IT IS 1999. The looming millennium is working Britain into a tizzy, but I have bigger concerns.

I'm standing in our school auditorium looking at a middle-aged woman holding a clipboard. She is sitting in one of the red theater seats fifteen rows back from the stage. Her eyeglasses are resting on her nose, and she is looking down, writing furiously.

I've been waiting a long thirty seconds. She nods. I take it as a sign to begin, and I start to speak. Silently, like some ferocious mime artist, she holds up the palm of her hand for me to stop. The whisper of a sound escapes and I close my mouth. I shuffle my feet, and the noise echoes cruelly around the empty auditorium.

I try to channel Julie Walters. I'm remaking her character from the film *Educating Rita*. I can hear her Liverpudlian accent in my head. I know I can't do it justice. I resolve to stick with what I have. Accents are not part of the grade. There's no point in trying and looking foolish. I can still get an A if I talk normally. Can I do that?

I look back up at the examiner. She is one of the most intimidating women I have ever set eyes on. She looks like she might have taken down Margaret Thatcher in a fight for her wardrobe.

I desperately start running over the lines in my head. I forget the second sentence. I silently curse myself. The voice is getting louder in my head. He is telling me what a fool I am. I can never be an actress. I can't do this. In a matter of seconds I'll humiliate myself. The horror is imminent. But there is still time to run. Run. Do it. Go.

I glance backwards for a second to judge the distance to the exit. But I stay glued to the stage floor. I can't let the stutter win. I can't give it that satisfaction. Angry determination seeps up through my legs, through my chest, and floods my brain.

I have no idea what will happen when I open my mouth, but I can't stay silent. I know that I won't run because if I run, the stutter has taken over. If that happens, all hope is gone. So I cross my fingers behind my back and start to make desperate pleas to a god I'm not sure I believe in. Just let me make it through this, let me be fluent. I'll do anything, I'll . . .

"Ready?"

She sounds bored, indifferent. It makes her even more petrifying.

I shuffle for a moment. She is looking at her notes and

intermittently peering at me from the top of her half-moon spectacles. Nervous energy bathes me in adrenaline. I'm made fluid by it. I start speaking, and the words come spewing forth,

"But I don't want to be myself." At first I don't believe my luck. The gamble has paid off. I force myself to stay calm, not to allow myself to be tricked by such early glory.

"Me? What's me? S s s some stupid woman who gives us all a laugh because she thinks she can learn, because she thinks one day she'll be like the rest of them, talking seriously, confidently, with knowledge, livin' a civilized life."

In spite of myself, in spite of Rita's bitter words, I'm euphoric. It is how speaking should be; rhythmic and expressive and indescribably easy. My tiny stumble barely registers. I start to move across the stage, embracing Rita's verbose, determined character. I can do her passion justice; I can make my voice reflect all the emotions trapped in my body. I am focusing so hard on remembering my lines, on marrying my gestures and the rhythm of my delivery, that I have almost, *almost* forgotten that I stutter.

As the final line approaches, time has morphed and buckled. I imagine that I have been speaking for ten minutes, but it could have been anything from five to fifty. I feel disconnected from myself, from reality. I relish the strangeness of it all. I feel how each fluent advance strengthens my confidence, how every successful line pushes my stutter further away. I balloon into my new persona until, at the end, I'm breathless and high. I'm victorious.

Unaware and profoundly unmoved by my metamorphosis, the examiner nods curtly and starts writing.

In the silent wake of my monologue I let myself believe the impossible. Perhaps this time it has gone away. Perhaps, through pure force of will, I have won the battle for good. I contemplate what that would feel like. What I would be if I didn't stutter.

"Name?" Her curt voice shatters my thoughts.

It takes me off guard and I feel the familiar desperation start licking around my nervous system. Instantly my defenses are weakened and made redundant. I know I'll be exposed.

"KKKK K K K K KK K K K ka ka ka ka ka ka kath kath erine."

The stutter has ravaged my name and, for the first time, I have her attention. It is undivided now. I'm not the average, precocious teenager that she had conjured in her head. Not the average teenage girl that she examines week after boring week.

"Katherine Preston?"

I nod.

"Katherine, is this your fifth acting exam?" There's a surprised intonation to her voice.

I nod again, "Yes, it is."

"Why did you choose a monologue?"

Cunning. It is not exactly the kind of question that warrants a nod or a two-word response.

The truth is that I have a greater chance of fluency with a monologue. There is none of the dangerous back-and-forth banter of dialogue. I am also the only one on the stage. If I embarrass myself, we are the only ones that will know. I'm not dragging anyone else down with me. If I'm going to lose the battle, I'm doing it silently with as few fatalities as possible.

That is the truth of the matter, but she doesn't need to know all of that.

"I find monologues stretch m m m m m my skills." This is not going to be pretty. I slide my hands into my pocket and pinch the top of my leg in desperation. I smile up at her as confidently as I can, "They force me to rr r r rely on no one bbb b b bbb but myself. They ch ch ch ch challenge me to learn a large swathe of m m m m material by heart."

I have lost all respect for my broken words. I don't want to incriminate myself anymore. Yet I want her to see that I have an intelligent answer for her, that I'm not some incoherent blubbering idiot.

She nods slowly as I speak, but her eyes give her away. They are transfixed on me. She's shocked. I am used to the shifting expressions, but they still bother me. The horrid surprise of stuttering.

I suspect that she is questioning what a girl with such an obvious stutter is doing acting. I hope she doesn't decide to turn into a dime-store psychologist. She looks like she might for a moment, but she says nothing. Nor do I.

In the years since my first disastrous attempt at speech therapy I have become adept at hauling my stutter around with me like a giant white elephant. I don't talk about it and nor does anyone else. I shout at my mum to silence any painful mention of it and never mention it to any of my friends. I'm pretending that my stutter doesn't exist and getting on with my life in the best way I can. I have adopted denial, and I'm clinging to it like a lifeline. If I don't talk about my stutter, maybe no one else will, maybe we will all just magically forget about it.

She looks at me for a moment. Her whole persona has changed, and the armor of the examiner has been chipped away. She seems softer when she speaks, "Thank you, Katherine. Your rendition was very, um, very impressive. Very . . . courageous."

Courageous, strong, determined. One of those euphemisms for "you have a severe disability and you are still living your life." Well done, you.

I thank her and walk out of the first set of double doors, wondering what she would have said if I hadn't stuttered. Would she have tactfully told me that my acting was utter rubbish? Who knows? I suspect that my stutter has just secured me a pity vote. I'm proud and repulsed at once.

FROM THE age of nine, I took on my stutter like a woefully incompetent soldier. Unfortunately, my stutter was a wily opponent. He encamped himself in my body and ensured that my personal battlefield was always in flux. "He" took me off guard, tricked me with moments and hours of fluency. He waited till I got cocky and then sneaked up with a guerrilla attack. Every time I opened my mouth, I was at his mercy. If I didn't hate him so much, I'd congratulate him for his effective manipulation. He was a much better fighter than I was.

At the time I believed that my stutter and I were somehow separated, that he and I were the two forces competing within my body. I never entertained the thought that he was part of me, that I was at war with myself. Instead, I found ways to counterattack, to try to thwart him. I knew that if I didn't open my mouth, my disability was hidden. Not just markedly less obvious or only obvious to the discerning viewer. No, it was completely and utterly disguised in silence. Mute, I was normal.

I have heard of stutterers who have chosen to be mute for years on end and have come out of their self-enforced silence with a surprisingly intact speaking voice. I find their stories fascinatingly at odds with my own experience. I always found that silence was lonely and debilitating in a way that was far sadder than the desperate fight of stuttering. I would rather risk the gauntlet of my speech, rather stutter and face the inevitable reaction. Silence reminded me of being alone: it made me feel as if I were trapped outside of the world by my stutter. When I sat on the edge of a conversation and said nothing, I felt beaten by it, as if the world was passing me by, and I was little more than an impotent spectator. I felt on the edge of invisibility.

Hiding was not sustainable, at least not for me. Despite my stutter I never liked solitude. I always craved being around others, always felt rejuvenated by their company, and I needed my voice to make people want to be around me. I needed it to whisper secrets to my friends, to make my cousins laugh, to ask for directions, to tell my parents that I loved them. I knew from a young age that communication was not all about our voices. Out of necessity I quickly learnt the beauty in the words I could speak with only a touch or a look. I could see the power of so-called nonverbal communication. But, in the end, it all came back to speech. Speech was the bedrock, the fundamental piece of our nature as human beings.

"What distinguishes us from apes is verbal language," explains the author David Shields. "If you are having trouble with that part of yourself, at its worst, it can make you feel scarily inhuman. You feel like you're part human and part monster." As a child that was how I felt. I felt not fully human.

I worshipped language. I watched how others spoke with obsessive, jealous interest. I watched strangers tell jokes on the Underground, I listened as parents told off their children and girlfriends shared the latest office gossip. I saw how they bandied their words about so carelessly, so constantly. I saw how they used their easily won language to console each other, to play, to argue, to shout opinions across a table. I saw what language came down to, what it really meant to me. It was intimately tied up with our need to connect, to voice our opinions, and to make a mark in the world.

Speech therapy was ruled out as an option. After my first failed attempt at the Michael Palin Centre I had gone back to the therapists, head hung low, to ask for help. Later I had gone to see a quiet speech therapist at a dingy National Health Service office after school. And yet none of it helped. I was always fluent in the speech therapy room as she told me to slow down and read long lists of words aloud. Yet I never wanted to slow down, I never wanted to compromise, and my stutter always came roaring back the next day as I launched into conversations at school. Eventually I swore off therapy, I swore that I would not put myself, or my parents, through the emotional turmoil anymore. I strategized, and I came up with a new form of attack to pull myself out of the silence. Denial.

I believed that it was just the method I had been searching for so desperately.

It was so beautifully simple. I would just pretend that I didn't stutter. I would pretend that I sounded like everyone else. I would brush away any mention of my stutter, treat it like a minor nuisance, and push forward regardless. The stutter would not rule my life. I would do anything and everything that a fluent person could do. I would suppress my own feelings in the hope that if I didn't speak about them, they would simply cease to be true.

So, as a teenager, I returned to my previous confidence with a vengeance. It was easy, unnervingly so. We were all pretending in our own ways, we were all pretending to be cool, to be confident, to have it all together. I loved to talk, and I loved to listen. I had a million opinions that I wanted to share, and I refused to be cowed by this "thing" I couldn't control. Luckily, underneath it all, I was pretty confident. I had the unerring optimism of my dad and the straightforward self-belief of my mum. I couldn't go too far wrong.

My stutter didn't change, but my acting skills certainly improved. I reentered the noisy bustle of the real world. I put my hand up in class, I slipped back into conversations, and I jumped back into games with my friends. I spoke readily, but I was still afraid of my stutter. I believed that the stutter was a red target on my back, and I knew that I had to up my game if I was going to survive. Determined to do anything not to expose my "real" voice, I took note of any chinks that I could see in my stutter's armor and devised some tactics to mask my voice.

Tactic number one was choosing my moments to speak.

I would not jump in wantonly. I noticed that my stutter was disabled if I spoke at the same time as others. So, if I wanted to jump into a group conversation, I would wait for the moment to strike. I learnt how to time the end of someone's speech, the moment when they were running out of breath and ramping up to their closing argument. While their words were trailing away, I would clamber to their last syllables. In a move that would make etiquette guru Lucie Clayton squirm in her twin set, I would ruthlessly cut them off and begin my sentence. They might look a little put out, but they wouldn't say anything. It was small enough to be a buzzing annoyance, but nothing they could really hold against me.

Tactic number two was a tad more tricky. It was less manageable and had more potential to humiliate me. I didn't stutter if I spoke in an accent. Few stutterers do. Later in my life, the actress Emily Blunt told me that she remembered her speech changing when her drama teacher encouraged her to do a play in a northern accent. She had grown up "tripping on certain words," but her stutter had become more forceful and, by the age of twelve, her mum had taken her to everything from cranial osteopathy to relaxation classes to try and help. Much like Samuel L. Jackson, Emily believed acting allowed her to be someone else for a while, to escape from the misjudgment of others. She believes that she rose to the occasion because of her teacher's confidence in her ability. In her words, "It was like a record skipping. If I could stop it, even momentarily, then that was a big deal. I felt confident that I could try it again in my everyday life."

Unfortunately, accents were never my strong suit, and they

were far from a breakthrough for me. All I had was a comedy Indian, a gimmicky posh British, and a slew of other made-up tonal variations. Telling a joke in an accent was fine, but it was more tricky to slip into a slightly insulting impersonation of a Glaswegian when I was simply asking someone how their day had been. I had to resume my regular voice eventually; I always knew that I couldn't keep up the pretense indefinitely. Even if I had possessed a smidgen of a talent for accents, I was certain that as soon as I got comfortable with a new voice, I would start stuttering. Perhaps, unlike Emily, I could never make myself believe that acting, or becoming someone else, was any kind of a cure. Instead, I stubbornly assumed that it was just the surprise of a new way of speaking that rendered me "fluent." I knew my stutter, and I knew that he was not so easily deceived. I knew that he would come storming back as soon as he was no longer distracted.

I had a third tactic up my sleeve. Having always been an avid reader, I collected words like my grandpa collected stamps. I filed each one away, labeled it in a certain context, so I could pull it out at a moment's notice. I taught myself how to become a gymnast in the game of word substitution. As soon as I could see the "danger words" looming ahead, or feel the nerves licking around my tongue, I would find a way to turn my sentence around or simply replace a needlessly challenging word. In the words of the author Benson Bobrick, I became an "ambulatory thesaurus." My words ran from the reasonable to the ridiculous. "Car" became more specifically "the Peugeot" or more pedantically "the auto." When I was feeling particularly cool, I believed I could even slip into my "ride." Telling my friends' parents that my mum was going to "swing by and pick me up in her ride" any second, that she was just caught up "buying some provisions for the kitchen" may have elicited some raised eyebrows in the school parking lot, but at least they didn't hear me stutter.

I enjoyed it, at first. I liked the sensation that I was winning, that I could dodge a block or repetition at a second's notice. But gradually I started to edit myself so heavily that my sentences became dangerously complicated, my descriptions overly obtuse. I lost control as my spoken sentences drifted dangerously away from the voice in my head. I began to see land mines everywhere, dotted across the horizon of my sentence so thickly that I couldn't say one word fluently. Simple questions turned into minefields for myself and my trapped audience. Even as a child, the actor Michael Palin remembers seeing that his father had so much to say, so many thoughts that he wanted to express and couldn't. "He would come out with a word which I knew wasn't the word he wanted to use." Michael remembers how he wanted to ask him to say it again, to say what he wanted rather than what he could, "but life isn't like that, and you move on rather quickly."

My speech took on a circuitous bent, and my seeming lack of memory made me act like a long-winded geriatric quizzing my listener. When asked where I went to school, I was not tempted to take on the challenge of the *Q* or the harsh wall of the *C* in Queen Anne's Caversham. Rather than be tripped up, I would mysteriously reply, "the school up the hill from Reading, no, not that one, the one that wears the cloaks, no the other one, yes, the one that's all girls." Most of the time I tried to pull it off with an ironic smile, as if I was perpetually part of some very private joke that only I understood.

My final tactic, the most long-lasting and sensible of my approaches, came down to choosing comrades whom I could trust. I was never after acquaintances, never after flighty friends to pass the time with. I steered clear of anyone spiteful or boring. I always surrounded myself with people whom I trusted, people who were intelligent and boisterous and loyal. I sought out people with open and generous faces.

Like many stutterers, I quickly realized that I needed only one person to feel less lonely, to feel accepted. Electrical engineer Nick Richard remembers feeling horribly ostracized in sixth grade. He remembers being miserable and be made to feel like a freak, and he remembers the day that changed. By the seventh grade he was already jaded, accustomed to the sound of sniggers behind his back and mockery to his face when he answered a question in class. "I was in math class, and the teacher asked us to show our homework on the board and explain it. I was used to being laughed at, but this one day there was this girl and she cheered for me after I finished." He smiles at the memory, "The first time it happened, I was really pissed, because I thought it was just a new level of insult. But she carried on doing it, and I started to realize that she appreciated my making the effort and actually doing it rather than cutting corners." He remembers how the experience changed him, how it gave him strength to form other friendships.

Claire was my oldest friend. I had known her for most of my memorable life. We fought like sisters, wore matching outfits for nearly a year, and had been inseparable since we were three years old. My army began with the two of us and grew from there. There was Soraya, another only child who had the sharpest sense of humor I knew. She was funny, stomach-achingly funny, but I was wary of her for a long time. I met her when I was five and spent a couple of years scared of her, not sure if we were friends, not sure whether to join forces or run away. I suspected that my stutter could be ample fodder for her sarcastic one-liners. Gradually, I learnt that I need not have worried. She proved to be one of my best friends and one of my most ardent supporters. There was a whole gang of us who stayed at each other's houses every weekend, who went on holidays together, and staged complicated musicals in Claire's basement.

Just before my eleventh birthday, my family decided to leave our home in London and move to the countryside. The move might have severed my friendships, it might have left me heartbroken for all the people I had to leave behind. Instead, three of us left London at the same time. Claire, Soraya, and I all moved to houses within driving distance of one another. By coincidence, or desperate persuasion, we all ended up as day girls at the same boarding school.

Over the next few years we fought, grew apart, and grew back together with a new group of friends. We gravitated towards people who were warm, loud, independent, and fearless. The kind of people who laughed loudly and were always up for mischief. They were all people who I wanted to be around, the type of girls I hoped to be, on my best days.

They became great friends, friends who had seen each

other morph from playful adolescence to burgeoning adulthood. We were mostly day girls, but Queen Anne's was pri-
marily a boarding school, so we were in our uniforms from
early morning chapel to home time at six thirty. We spent
more time with each other than with anyone else. We became
each other's family, the sort of friends who told each other
anything and everything. Well, almost anything.

We never spoke about my stutter. They took their lead
from me, and I silently thanked them for it. We teased each
other relentlessly but no one ever touched on the loaded territory of my speech. I wasn't a "stutterer" in their eyes, and
I loved them for that. I was just Katherine, or Kat, as I grew
older. I wasn't one of the people who had something wrong
with them. I was part of the "in" crowd.

I have learnt that I was lucky, that lots of stutterers are made
to feel like a traveling freak show, there for the benefit of others' amusement. I was never bullied outright. I fended off the
odd insult or damning laughter, but nothing that could break me
down systematically. However, I know of kids who were bullied,
laughed at, and mocked mercilessly. Gerard Enright, a retired
NYC Teamster, remembers growing up as a stutterer and attend-
ing the speech therapy class at his school. Over sixty years later,
he still calls it a "hell on earth" where the jocks would stand by
the windows in the back wall "and make faces with their hands
clasped around their necks." He tried to stand up for the girls
who stuttered by taking on the whole football team and "got a
whipping" every week.

My childhood was idyllic in comparison, but I always
worried that I might be discovered at some point. I was se-

cretly afraid that I would be found out, that someone would let on that I stuttered, that I was not really all that cool. There were enough spiteful girls in my school, enough potential bullies, to make me believe that my secret might be laid bare at any moment. So I formed a shield of friends who would protect me. Today I suspect that they barely realized how they ordered for me in restaurants, how they introduced me to new people so I didn't have to say my name, how they let me slip away at just the right moments.

With or without knowing it, they became my bodyguards, my protection against the world. It was their faith in me— their insistence that I come along to every party, that I go on holidays, that I learn how to ride horses—that fortified me. It was their steadfast friendship and my parents' love that gave me the strength that carried me throughout my life. With my arms looped through theirs, I felt safe. Yet I knew that they would not always be around, I knew that I had to do every-thing in my power to erase the x that I thought my stutter might still be drawing on my back.

At school I was always running away from anything that would "out" me as a "stutterer." I tried to excel in every field I could, to shine the spotlight towards my accomplishments and away from my disappointing speech. If I couldn't be the best speaker, then at least I would try to make myself the best friend, the best student, the best daughter that I could be. I was fiercely loyal to anyone I loved and always on the lookout for a new way to prove myself. I quickly saw that the ath-letic girls at school were always popular, always well liked. So I tried lacrosse and netball and gymnastics. I was terrible.

I liked swimming, but as my body began to balloon in strange places, the appeal of squeezing into a Lycra swimsuit lessened significantly. Musicians seemed to be cool, so I took up playing the drums. My left hand dragged behind awkwardly, never quite as dexterous as my right, however much I willed it to cooperate. I took up art. It was not quite as cool as music or sports, but I loved it. I loved the creation of it, the quiet, the option to erase it all and start again. There was something pleasantly honest and elemental about drawing, and I felt at ease amidst the weirdly wonderful characters of summer art school.

I was not alone in wanting to compensate. I know of other stutterers who joined every sports team at their school, who did solos for their choir, who won every prize on the debate team. Unknown to each other, we were all driven by a determination to succeed in other areas, to let our singing voice or our game playing do the talking for us. As the basketball player Bob Love remembers, "All through high school, people laughed at me. It got so bad that I had to laugh with them to keep from crying. But I was lucky, I could play sports. I could hide a lot of that hurt on the basketball courts and the football field. I was a pretty good athlete, and you could lose yourself in sports and forget about your stutter, forget about your problems."

What do you do if, despite all your best attempts, you can't outrun or outmaneuver the bullies? What do you do if people stand on your feet when you try to talk or pick a fight with you just because you seem an easy target? From all the kids I have spoken to, it seems that boys face outright physical bullying more frequently than girls. Afraid of being teased, or reeling from the punches of too many bullies, lots of boys bulk up. They quickly learn how to throw a punch, how to let their muscles and their fists do the speaking for them. Sweet-natured lifeguard Matt Murray bottled up all of his anger until he took up mixed martial arts as a way of venting his frustration. He earned his black belt in Brazilian Jujitsu when he was only eighteen, has dislocated every joint in his body at least once, and has ended up in hospital a few times. Much like Matt, Jake Steinfeld was cruelly teased and mocked as a child. Having been nicknamed the "t-t-t-typewriter" by his classmates because of his repetitive style of speech, Jake went on to become a Hollywood body builder, daring anyone to taunt him.

I never had to perfect my right hook. Instead, in the rigorously academic atmosphere of my school, I compensated for my stutter by getting the best grades possible. My parents and my teachers encouraged me; they never doubted me, never saw my stutter as any kind of a hindrance. Within the school's walls my stutter was never given any air time. The classrooms provided the neatly black-and-white world that I wanted in the rest of my life. If I worked hard at something, my grades would reflect the effort. I wrote the best essays I could, forced my reluctant mind around complex math equations, and took up drama and debate with the determined conviction of someone who knows that she had something to prove to the world.

It wasn't always easy to break free of the stuttering label, but it felt necessary. I believed that I had to do well academically if I was going to survive, if I was going to join all my friends in the inevitable march towards university and beyond. I knew that I had to be likeable, I had to be fun to spend time around so that people would want to be around me in spite of my speech.

Luckily, by the age of fifteen, my friendships felt unbreakable. Hiding my stutter and fighting against it had secured good friends, strong grades, and praise from my family. It got me everything I wanted, but there were times when it just didn't cut it. Times when, for all my acting and pretending that I was just like everyone else, my "true" nature revealed its ugly head.

WE ARE sitting in the classroom, waiting for our teacher to arrive. We are sprawled over the furniture, five of us sitting on the small wooden tables with our scuffed Dr. Martens on the floor and our feet tapping on the chairs. Amey is balancing precariously on the warping back legs of her chair. All six of us are talking at once. It is Monday morning, and we have a few stolen minutes before class begins to recount the weekend's excitement. Later the stories will stretch over scribbled notes and whispered secrets, but right now they are fresh and recalled breathlessly.

Monday morning is typically the best day of the week, and today is better than most. Today we have something *big* to talk about. By some miracle Claire's parents had allowed her to throw a house party over the weekend. In a move that made them the coolest parents on the planet, they had discreetly slipped out at seven on Saturday night with the promise that they'd be back by midnight. There were a few passing shots from her dad: "Don't touch my liquor cabinet, call us if there are any problems, no one let the dog out, stay out of our bedroom." We heard him, sort of. We were too excited getting ready to pay too much heed. The Smirnoff ices were chilling in the fridge as we touched up the last of our makeup.

Weeks earlier we had invited everyone that we liked in our year at school and called up our friends at the nearby all-boys' school. By the time eight rolled around, there were at least thirty of us strewn around the house. At the time I remember feeling silly in my outfit. I remember worrying that I didn't look as thin or sexy as everyone else. But by Monday morning, I had forgotten all of that. The night had become "epic," "hilarious," "the best party so far." Hindsight had gilded it and made it glorious, better than it could have ever hoped to be on the actual night.

"What about when Andi spotted Tom drinking Wally's 1984 merlot?" chimes in Amey.

"Or when Paul went missing for three hours and we sent out a search party into the fields?" counters Liz.

"And we found him asleep in my parent's bathroom," sighs Claire in mock exasperation. Paul is her boyfriend, and she is the only one of us to have a fully fledged boyfriend. She starts giggling again, "What about when I slipped down the stairs and tumbled all the way down before hitting Giles and landing on her at the bottom."

"We all know what happened next." I can't resist. It is too good a story not to tell and I'm having such a great time reliving the night. I have been imagining the delivery in my head since we started talking. But now I have their eager attention, all of them. The excitement of our conversation has bled out to the rest of the classroom, to all the quieter boarders who had not been able to escape for the weekend. The room is now silent apart from our storytelling, all eyes staring in our direction. I never liked having an audience.

"While Claire was wrapped in ice packs after her tumble"— I throw in some finger quotations for effect. The "tumble" may or may not have been booze induced.

I'm drawing it out. Planning the punch line in my head.

"—the r r rest of us were in pandemonium downstairs."

Nothing to break the flow of the story, just a minor glitch. I don't let it derail me. I still have the momentum I need, "We could hear a hissing sound. And then someone shouted GAS!"

I'm on a real roll now. I am speaking louder, speeding up the pace of my delivery, "So anyone with a cigarette starts bolting towards the fields. We're convinced the house is about to launch into an inferno." I pause for effect, "Then I started running up the stairs. I'm shouting at everyone that we have a gas leak, telling them to go outside. It's 11:45. The parents will be back soon. So I slip rushing up the stairs and I burst into Claire's room. And I deliver the bad news that Armageddon is about to ensue. And she looks at me. Aghast."

The moment is here, the punch line is upon me. They're all looking at me. Bugger. I have to get it out. I can't let myself down. I'm approaching the glory of the finish line. I can't fumble now.

"So she looks at me and says, 'But we don't h h h h h h h h h h h.'" Shit. I'll run up at it again. I still have their attention. "We don't h ha ha ha ha ha ha ha ha."

I'm losing them. I can see it. They're good friends, they won't abandon me, but I can feel that I'm losing them in the carnage of my delivery. I look around the room and see two girls look at each other and smirk. Later one of them will end up in jail and the other will disappear into some mediocre oblivion, but at that moment they are mean and spiteful in the way that only pretty teenage girls can be.

I feel foolish. But I can't give up. "But we don't ha ha ha haaaa." I'm stretching it out. Willing the word to come: "have, we don't have gas."

"But we don't have gas!" I spit it out, finally intact. But it's too late.

My friends smile and then they laugh. But we all know that the rhythm of the joke was stretched too far, it went saggy and broke on me.

Amey retells the last line. And we laugh again. It really is pretty funny. Just not when I tell it. My stutter decimates the punch line. As always.

No one says anything. We carry on telling stories. Later that day I have forgotten the incident. Well, almost. I tell myself that it really wasn't all that important. It wasn't the end of the world. But it chipped away at me. Deep inside me it left an imprint that I couldn't easily erase.

CHAPTER 5

ART OF FLIRTING

IT IS MARGINALLY less glamorous than I had envisaged, but the sticky-floored, pop-pumping world of Reading's nightlife has been opened to me. I have looked the gargantuan bouncers in the eye and passed the test without being asked for my ID. I shimmy victoriously down the psychedelically patterned carpet.

Greedily I inhale the smell of stale cigarette smoke. I can see Soraya and Liz already pushing their way forward at the throbbing bar. The others are on their way. I catch Liz's eye and bring my cupped hand back and forth to my face mouthing, "Bacardi Breezer" as I point to the alcopop of choice in another punter's hand. She smiles and gives me a thumbs-up.

Now I just have to stake out a spot for us. We will migrate to the dance floor later, but it is still early and only a handful of confident, or heavily inebriated, girls are swaying across the UV-lit playpen. I feel seductively grown-up as I walk on my own around the bar, searching for an empty table. There are no chairs in Bar Oz, so I lean against the table and attempt to ooze mystery.

I start to worry that my jeans are too tight. I haven't yet lost my euphemistically termed "puppy fat." I tug upwards on my belt loop and shift my weight from one high heel to the other. The soles of my new shoes stick suspiciously to the carpeted floor. I bought them this morning and worry that I may already be losing feeling in my big toe. I chalk it up as another great milestone on the way to becoming a woman.

Lost in my thoughts I glance up to see a boy looking at me. He's on the other side of a large group, but every time they shift, his eyes appear again. I don't know what to make of it. I have been to an all-girls' schools since the age of four. We have a gang of friends at the nearby all-boys' school, but they are just "the boys." Boys in bars are still a new breed to me.

Recently it feels as if my hormones have taken my body hostage. I have gone from finding boys repulsive to deciding that they are endlessly fascinating. I'm sure that all manner of thoughts must have taken up space in my brain before, but now there is precious little room for anything else. Kissing boys, being kissed by them, worrying about why I'm not being kissed by them—it keeps me busy for hours.

Nervously I hazard a glance back in his direction. This time he smiles slightly. Having spent an hour getting ready at Claire's house earlier, I am relieved that all the hard work has not gone to waste. I smile back gratefully.

It is foolish and I know it. I blame my hormones because the sane part of me is terrified. Quickly I look away again. This time I see a bit of movement in my peripheral vision. He's on the move. I practically beckoned him over. My heart starts pounding. I silently plead for my friends to join me because I need backup and quick. Too late. He's two paces away. Stuck to the floor, I watch him slide between the final two girls and demolish the safe distance between us.

"Hi." He has to shout to make himself heard over the blaring voices of Destiny's Child. "My name's John."

"Hi," I scream back. He smells of Lynx and sweat, and the drag of his last cigarette is still lingering on his breath.

"I saw you from over there." In case I had forgotten, he points over to his group of friends. They laugh and wink on cue.

"Yes." I'm stalling, still hoping that the girls will arrive in time.

"What's your name?"

I look at him for a second. His eyes are wide, open, trusting. His body is leant consciously towards me, his bare forearm touching mine. I decide to dodge the question.

"Wouldn't you like to know."

It seems to work. He smiles and leans in closer. His cheek touches mine as he whispers in my ear, "Well, I would. That's why I asked you."

This is not award-winning flirting. I sound like the beginning of some poorly scripted porn movie. I lean away from him, too aware of the way my heart has started pounding, too aware of the heat licking up my body. I have to get onto firmer ground. I don't want to risk my name, not yet, not until

I have a drink in my hand. I want to preserve whatever image he has of me at that moment. I want to maintain the illusion that I am confident, alluring, easily flirtatious. Fluent. I want to preserve his fantasy of me.

"It's Samantha." The lie comes all too easily. It tramples on my game and deflates my interest.

"Amanda?"

Sure. Samantha, Amanda. I don't care, I'll take it. I'm bored by myself and by him. Frustrated by the echo of my foolishness. The guy has no chance. I can't start a relationship, or whatever this is, by lying about something as elemental as my name, "Yup, Amanda."

Then, with impeccable timing, the cavalry arrives. They all bundle around the table at once. Giggling girls clasping alcopops victoriously. They notice him as they hand over my drink. As Amey starts nudging me, I desperately wish that he wasn't standing there with that stupid grin on his face. I want to get away from him before he unveils my new pseudonym.

I keep my distance and bring the bottle up to my lips as I turn back to him, "Hey, I'm going to catch up with the girls. I'll see you a little later." It is a cold brush-off, but I can't imagine that he will take much offense. He looks put out for a second, and I fear that I've underestimated him. I watch his smile buckle, and after a few long seconds, he nods and walks off. The girls start teasing me. All is back to normal.

Two drinks down, we're on the dance floor. I watch John whispering in some other girl's ear. I watch her giggle in response, and I turn away before I catch his eye. I dance until my feet have grown blisters on every toe, until I can feel sweat dripping down my spine. I finally leave the floor when the DJ decides to spin Gareth Gates's latest single. Gates is the runner-up in England's first *Pop Idol.* I had voted for the other guy, voted for anonymity, but living rooms around England are still marveling at the nervous, stuttering Gates who turned melodically fluent when he started singing. In breathy tones, morning television hosts are still talking about the miraculous phenomenon.

As much as I hate the fact that stuttering is suddenly in vogue, as much as I loathe the fact that I can't turn on the radio without some earnest presenter explaining to listeners that no one stutters when they sing, they have a point. I know that I'm just bitter. I am practically tone-deaf so, unless singing involves a shower or a very loud stereo system, it is out of the question. Luckily, dancing is a pretty decent alternative. When I dance, my whole body becomes my voice. I can be sexy and silly and confident without saying a single word; smiles and hand gestures more than suffice. My body may not be perfect, but it moves how I want it to, and doesn't abandon me on a whim.

Having been forced off the dance floor by Gates's crooning, I need another release. I start to make my way to the bar to buy the next round. I slide between oily bodies and push forward to get the barman's attention.

"Hey, I saw you dancing out there. What's your name?" His face is beading with sweat and his hair is standing upright in crisp gelled peaks as he leans on the bar next to me. This time I'm ready for it, I won't be flummoxed again, "K At."

"Hat?"

Hat. Really?

"No, no. Kat." I pause for a minute. He still looks con-fused. I'm concerned that his next guess may be "Fat" so I jump in quickly, "It's Kat. Like the a a a a a a a a a animal." Before I can stop myself, I do a clawing action with my hand, in case he has never heard of this rare animal, a cat.

He laughs, "Are you drunk? You're slurring your words."

My natural confidence instantly deflates, "No. I'm not drunk. I ss s s s ss s s stutter."

I smile, to mitigate the stutter, perhaps to apologize, to keep him interested.

"What?"

I think about screaming my reply at him again. Unsurpris-ingly I don't. "Never mind."

"You have such a soft voice. I can barely understand." I have already started turning away when he makes his final attempt. "You're cute, though."

"CUTE." A four-letter word, a poor consolation prize when you're aiming for sexy and alluring. I was "cute" in spite of my stutter or because of it. A compliment born out of pity. "Cute" like some inebriated teddy bear propping up the bar. It was not the sophisticated look I was aiming for. It pushed me back down the ladder a few rungs, regressed me dangerously back towards floral dresses and velvet headbands.

My stutter had always made men see me in a certain way. Not always, I suppose. There had certainly been men who laughed or walked away or looked at me in plain disgust, but there were always the others in their wake. I knew that, because of my speech and my blond hair and my height, I was typically seen as someone who needed protection. It helped, in its way. But it was dangerous, too. I felt like I let people down. Because I was not always what they expected; I was not the damsel in distress that they may have been looking for. I was grumpy, I laughed loudly, I was stubborn and opinionated and spontaneous. I loved to be protected, but I was looking for someone I could protect as well, someone who could stand up to me, someone who saw me as his equal.

Although my apparent cuteness mitigated certain things for me, I saw it as yet another hurdle to overcome on my way to becoming a fully fledged woman. There were lots of stumbling blocks ready to trip me up. Stuttering was just a part of the joyful obstacle course. Along with acne and weight fluctuations and emerging body parts, it was tied up in the hormonal party that made teenage life just that little bit more challenging. And the tricky business of womanhood wasn't purely physical. We also had to learn how to make ourselves interesting. We had to learn how to flirt.

As a woman I quickly realized that flirting was part of my arsenal. It was a survival skill. No one hands you a guidebook on your fifteenth birthday. They should. Instead, you just have to watch and learn. So I started to gather my proof. I watched movies, I read books, I took notes on the people around me. Women teased men, they told them jokes, they complimented them, they dropped mysteriously loaded questions. They were eloquent and witty and cutting and thoughtful. They spoke *a lot.*

I quickly came to the conclusion that speaking and flirting were inexorably linked. Men had it easier. They were allowed to grunt the odd reply or to take on the brooding, mysterious air of James Dean. As women, the burden of conversation was on us. I had seen the movies, I knew that candlelit dinners would lapse into awkward silences if we didn't take the reins.

So I devised a way around it, but it was a tricky maneuver. I had to learn to talk just enough to be intriguing while, imperceptibly, asking more than my share of questions. At first I came across like a Gestapo inquisitor, but I eventually improved. I would talk enough to ignite another's interest and then slip another broad question into the end of my sentence. I loved hearing stories and could keep another person talking for hours with a couple of prompts and weighty head nods. I would smile and laugh and frown at all the right moments. I would brush my hand against theirs or touch their arm as a signal to carry on. Slowly, I realized that it worked. People loved to talk about themselves, and they found something compelling about an avid listener. I had that role perfected. It was not entirely honest, because I was not venting my opinions or sharing my passions. But I decided that that could come later, that I needed to get a foot in the door first. Plus, I had a certain innate talent for listening. I enjoyed it, I was interested in everyone's stories, interested in hearing the longest tale they could tell. I could perfect the role of confidante and sounding board.

If the man in question was the quiet type, I had a backup. A slightly less than ideal plan B: alcohol. Any kind of booze. Beer, wine, spirits, it didn't matter. Drink anesthetized me against the apprehension of speaking, and I had an army of bottle-shaped wingmen waiting patiently for me behind the bar.

Sitting in a café in Los Angeles with Nora O'Connor, I realized that I was not the only one. As Nora put it, "When I picked up my first drink, it was like everything that I hated about myself, everything that I believed I wasn't going to be able to do, went away." I suspect that stutterers are not unique in this. I suspect that many teenagers welcome the opportunity to dull their hesitancies and leap forth without abandon. We want to be loud and funny and witty and carefree. We crave an escape. We all want a break from the monologue that is going on in our heads.

And yet addiction and escape have an even stronger allure for stutterers. The experience is not purely physiological. Drugs have a physical effect on our speech. Few stutterers are amphetamine abusers (substances like cocaine generally increase the level of stuttering), but alcohol and other drugs can lower our anxiety and make us temporarily fluent. It can smooth our syllables and allow us to present ourselves in the way we want. If alcohol or drugs dull the ache that stuttering leaves lingering in your body, the attraction is dangerously powerful. Today Nora O'Connor is a social worker working in a residential drug treatment program for male parolees in Los Angeles, but she remembers a time when she could not function without liquid confidence. "I dealt with my stutter by drink and then drugs. That was on a daily basis from the age of twelve. That was the way I was able to live in the world as opposed to something that would have been more drastic," she recalls. "I realize now that alcohol and drugs were able to save my life, but if I wasn't able to get into recovery I definitely would have ended up dead or incarcerated."

Luckily, the temptation of release offered by drugs or alcohol is tempered by a fear of being out of control. When we pitch power against fluency, the losses often outweigh the gains. For all my life, control, or the hope for control, largely had the upper hand. I wanted to be in charge, to have total mastery over my body. Stuttering took away quite enough of my control as it was. I wasn't inclined to lose any more of my faculties.

One glass of wine and I was pleasantly merry and a little more fluent: one glass was perfect. Yet one was never enough, it was too tempting to maintain the high. By two glasses, my stutter was more aggressive than before. By the third glass, I was approaching stumbling territory, but back to near-fluency. Three drinks down, and I was already regretting the first.

It was a fine line to tread. Today I can still see the appeal of not having to deal with my stutter. Not having to feel the words clawing to be free or to face my fear of rejection. Sober, I saw everything. I felt my own desperate desire to be liked, to be sought after. I watched my listeners' shifting expressions, the way my stutter froze their faces or carved lines in their foreheads. I heard their laughter and saw the backs of their shirts as they walked away. Whatever I wore, however

I painted my face, I was still a "stutterer." There was nothing that could cover up my voice for long.

So I learnt to use my stutter to my advantage. I got myself accepted at Durham University, part of England's unofficial "Ivy League" of prestigious universities. I arrived as a wide-eyed "fresher" as the group of friends that I had grown up with scattered to universities throughout the country. I had a blank slate to start from, and I decided that I needed a filter. Anyone who laughed at me once, who frowned, who looked away was mercilessly crossed off my Christmas list.

As the writer Ted Hoagland explains, "When I would go to a party and I would start to stutter, three out of four women would step back. Some were very rude and completely heartless, but in general they would not be unkind or rude, they would just step back because I was not someone who interested them. But one out of four would step closer. It didn't alarm them and they would step closer to listen. They would want to know what I was saying and who I was. Then quite magically, if they opened up to me, I would stutter less and less."

In many ways the technique works well. It weeds out the good and the bad, but it doesn't make the process any less terrifying. As much as I tried, I could never hide my stutter completely. I could just about accept that people could see me stuttering, but I was afraid of anyone finding out about the wealth of fear and insecurity that lay behind it.

University is a challenging time for many stutterers, for many people. It is the first time that you are pushed out of the safety of home. The first time that you have to constantly introduce yourself to make friends and carve out a social life. You have to speak up in seminars, answer questions in lectures, and tell stories in the college bars. Your stutter may have lain dormant at school only to be fueled by the fear of imminent academic and social embarrassment.

Cat was the first friend I made at Durham, the first person to sail through my bullshit filter. She was funny and kind, we had practically the same name and grew up in the same countryside town of Henley. We were two peas in a pod, almost. When I arrived at Durham I felt adrift, scared, and excited. Cat grounded me; she made it feel like home, made me feel like I had an instant family.

History repeated itself, and my friendships grew from there. She introduced me to her friends and I made my own. I sought out people who were funny, generous, intelligent, and crazy enough to meet every expectation I had of uni life. We had picnics in the shadow of the medieval castle, woke up to the ringing of the cathedral bells, carried library books up the cobbled streets, and stumbled out of formal dinners with our academic gowns trailing behind us through the courtyards. I spent the hours I should have been cramming for exams rehearsing complicated dance routines. My tolerance for cheap red wine soared, and I learnt to love the sound of Latin and the exclusivity of private jokes. For the first time in my life I had a nickname that stuck. Some people still called me "Kat," but my housemates dubbed me "Petit." They were teasing me for my height and nothing else, and I loved them for it.

I adored every moment of it, and yet it was the first time in my life that I felt truly intimidated by the people around me. I had worked hard to be accepted at Durham, and yet I was ill-prepared for the level of academic rigor or the amount of speaking required. I began to dread the seminar discussions and started to have heart palpitations in preparation for the fortnightly presentations. I worried that not speaking up in class discussions made me look less intelligent, or less engaged than everyone else around me. I had to work harder than ever before to keep up and to speak up. It was humbling and exhilarating to be around such intelligent people.

After years of life in an all-girls' school, it was the first time that I had classes with boys, the first time that men became my teachers. It was from my male friends that I learnt how to think like an historian, how to focus my brain enough to write essays after a night playing drinking games. It was boys who taught me to drink port, to like classical music, and to smoke pot. They showed me the joy I could feel being swung around the dance floor in a dress that swept behind me. I learnt to appreciate their honesty, their intellect, and their curious intensity. There was only one thing missing. Finding a bona fide "boyfriend" eluded me.

Until I met the South African. The South African leant in closer when I stuttered. When I met him on a night out, I stuttered ferociously on my name. In response he smiled, he never broke my gaze. He impressed me. Against all odds, he seemed to be attracted by my stutter.

"What do you think of my speech?" I slurred at him one drunken evening. I suspected that he was just indulging me, and alcohol made me dangerous.

"I think it makes you stronger," he answered without missing a beat.

If I had meant it as a test, he had passed.

"Strong" was better than "vulnerable" or "broken." Strong sounded positive at least. Strong was a giant leap forward from "cute." Strong, along with fierce and passionate, was how I wanted to see myself. Plus, by then, I was pretty outwardly strong. So was he, outwardly. Inwardly we were both a little battered and bruised. Everyone knew our secrets and no one spoke to us about them. I stuttered, and he was an orphan.

So I believed that we could heal each other. I wanted to help him. I wanted to fill up the gaping hole that had been cut in his life. My listening skills were finally being put to a real use. I could absorb all his horror stories, his nightmares, and his hopes. I could tie them to my own.

Perhaps it was not the ideal start to a relationship, but we fell in love, and I fell in love with the idea of us. I dreamed that a "real" relationship would somehow validate me. It would prove to everyone that I was loveable, that my stutter didn't turn me into a leper.

When we are well aware of our own weakness it can be all too tempting to tether ourselves to someone, to something, "normal." I know of a stutterer who married his wife because he thought that she might be the only person who could ever love him. I've met men and women who have never really been in love, who coupled themselves to the first person who didn't run away from their speech, the first person who endorsed them.

I went out with the South African because I knew he loved

me, because I loved him, and because I saw pieces of myself reflected in his hazel eyes. For the first few months it was too good to be true. There were midnight picnics and mini-breaks. Everyone told me that relationships were hard, that they required work. I scoffed at their naïveté. It was all so easy.

Then he graduated and took off to travel around the world. As much as I was glad for him, I cried bitterly when he left. Suddenly, the easy intensity of our relationship was replaced with anxiety and the dreaded curse of talking on the phone. The phone had never been my strong suit, and now the immediacy of my entire relationship depended on it.

On the phone all communication rests on our voices. Having a winning smile or a look of deep understanding does precious little to move the conversation forward. And so the stutterer is tested to her limit. There is a lot of repetition. You have no idea what is happening on the other side of the line. Where are they? Have you caught them at a good time? I tend to picture my listener as unduly impatient, tapping his fingers on the table with a hundred other more pressing commitments.

On the phone, the stutterer is up against some pretty powerful odds, and it is tempting to find ways around the problem. The singer Chris Trapper remembers developing a complex solution to his phone anxiety as a young guy who wanted to ask girls out on dates. "I would speak into a boom box and prerecord the introduction, 'Hi, is Jackie there, please?' I would dial, then push Play, then stop it. It would get me past that very panicky point." It worked wonders as long as no unexpected questions arose.

I met others who took an even more extreme approach and simply refused to talk on the phone at all. Morgan Maxwell, a self-employed real estate appraiser in Tucson, Arizona, remembers having a secretary for many years and telling her on her first day that "if she ever got me on the phone, I would fire her."

Apart from looking in the mirror, giving myself a friendly face to talk to, I never came up with any ingenious solutions. I just barreled forward, like always. I told myself and my housemates how excited I was about the nightly phone call from some static-filled phone in South America with a two-second delay and a dodgy echo. I was optimistic. I thought we could make it. I ignored how much I was starting to resent it, how much I was starting to resent him.

The phone didn't break us up, but it didn't exactly keep us together. He was gone for almost two years, and by the end of it our relationship had faltered and exhausted itself somewhere in the middle of the Atlantic Ocean. We tried to revive it in London, three years after we had first met, but by that point bitterness had tainted every memory.

When it finally died I decided to revisit the question I had asked years ago. Perhaps I was hoping for some final shred of hope, perhaps I wanted to finally ask the question that had kept me occupied through every long-distance phone call, perhaps I was simply masochistic. What did he really think of my stutter?

His reply came over a long email. It hadn't bothered him, he wrote. He had noticed it more with others, or after I came back from speech therapy, but it had never been a problem for him. I unclenched my toes as I read on, relieved. Then, in the middle, he started talking about his friends. He related their surprise that he would go out with someone who stuttered: "They assumed I would go for someone more conventionally perfect."

My world quickly became cold and still. My laptop screen brightened and bulged towards me. I could see myself, I could picture the frozen snapshot of my pale face huddled over the screen. It was not how I wanted to look, not the image I wanted to develop. That moment took its place amidst the worst times of my life.

Because I thought that he hadn't noticed. I had genuinely fooled myself into thinking that they all just saw beyond it. I thought I had talked enough, told enough jokes, worked out often enough to mitigate my stutter. I thought that I had sounded intelligent enough that we had all just skated over my speech together hand in hand. It turns out I was just the fool out there on my own.

He had confirmed my worst fears, confirmed that all the pretense was useless, confirmed that I was a "stutterer" in many people's eyes. Unintentionally, he had underlined it as a swearword, a weapon, and a dismissal. He had confirmed that I was broken and that my greatest weakness was visible for all to see. I was a pity case, a second prize in the grand girlfriend stakes.

Perfect. Perfect like a sexless, flawless Barbie doll? Perfect like all other girls in the college? The word echoed heavily around my brain and then came to rest. It wedged itself into my memories and festered there.

CHAPTER 6

ERECTING MY OWN GLASS CEILING

London, November 2006

I<small>T IS MY</small> foray into the workplace, and I have a six-foot beauty for a boss. Her legs tower skywards from the perspective of my sinking swivel chair. She leans against my desk and swishes her blond hair towards me as she tells me how her boyfriend is driving her mad because he keeps buying her flowers, as a joke. She hates them. Poor love.

"So there's a news conference tonight or an art gallery opening. Which would you rather cover?"

I try to look like she has posed a fascinating dilemma and I'm seriously contemplating my options. In reality, there is no chance that I'm choosing the conference. The very thought throws me into cold sweats. The idea of raising my hand and having to shout out a witty, pertinent, or cutting question at a jostling press junket sounds about as pleasant as having my hand sawn off with a blunt spoon.

Eventually I nonchalantly reply, "I'll take the art gallery. What's the story?"

"Rod Stewart should be there. He was just on *X Factor* as a guest judge, and we want to hear what he *really* thinks about the contestants."

I jot down some notes and nod furiously. "Got it!" A cutting exposé on Rod's hidden feelings about the singers. "Sounds fascinating." Yes, this is just the sort of compelling journalism that I had always dreamed of doing.

I jump in a taxi outside the office. I'm only an intern at the paper, but I hope the driver fancies that I am some hard-hitting journalist. I pull out my pad and try to perfect the world-weary look that I have seen other hacks adopting. I tell him the address as we wind our way through the rainy London streets.

I run over my questions and the latest news on Rod as we swerve through Knightsbridge and up Piccadilly. When we pull up in front of the swanky Soho gallery I realize that I have left my umbrella at the office. I run out of the taxi, coat draped over my head, trip on the pavement, and stumble towards the doorman, looking bedraggled, "I'm here with the *Telegraph*'s Society section." He looks suspicious for a moment and reluctantly unhooks the red rope.

Now I'm in, but I have no clue what to do next. The celebrities have not yet started arriving, so I have a moment to sip

champagne and take in the artwork. It seems to be a decon-
structionist take on the coat hanger.

"It's ugly as hell, isn't it?"

He has an East End accent, and I would peg him to be
somewhere in his early forties. I'm surprised to see a cravat at
his neck and a walking cane swinging from his hand.

"I'm not sure I'd take it that far."

"Oh, you know you would. You're just worried that the artist is wandering around somewhere." He pauses and I crack
a smile. He leans in. "Don't worry, she's not here yet; you can
be as honest as you like."

I like him instantly. I find out that he's a dealer. I tell him
that I interned at *Artforum* in New York for a couple of months
a year ago, and we banter for a while about the scene. I wonder if the evening will actually be a total laugh. By the time
he has introduced me to his boyfriend, I feel like I have been
initiated into some bohemian club.

Then I see Rod arrive. I take a final swig of bubbly and tell
my new best friend that I need to talk to someone.

I plan out the opening line in my head as I squeeze between
the partygoers. "Hi, Rod, I'd love to chat to you about your
recent cameo on *X Factor*." Or perhaps a more hard-hitting,
"Mr. Stewart, tell me, are all the *X Factor* contestants as horrendous as they look on the telly?"

By the time I get within two feet of him, I am hyperventilating. I start to circle him like some manic stalker. On my
third rotation, I have still not casually caught his eye, and I
am beginning to feel nauseous.

Finally, I stop pacing, take my place next to him, and tap

him on the shoulder. I instantly regret it. He turns around and looks at me coldly, "Hi, Rod." As it comes out of my mouth it already feels too familiar, too presumptuous. "Um, my name is, um, um, K K K K K Ka Ka." He looks at me and then glances around the room, like he's worried he's on some candid camera show. I ramp up to it again, "Katherine Preston." He looks a little relieved. "I'm here with the *Telegraph*—"

He starts to back away. "I don't want to talk. I'm just here to enjoy the artwork."

There is no anger to his voice, just stony resolve. To underline his point, he turns his back on me and resumes his previous conversation.

Embarrassed, I stand awkwardly next to him for a moment. When I finally slide away, I glumly wonder what on earth I'll say when I get back to the office in the morning without any sort of story to my name.

I wander back to my friend. I see that he has a group around him and contemplate walking in the other direction, but then I catch his eye and he beckons me over.

"Everyone, this is Katherine." They nod politely in my direction, mumble their names, and then resume a heated debate about the state of modern art. "What's wrong with you? You look miserable, darling."

I tell him about my boss, my job, why I'm at the exhibition and my horrid meeting with Rod.

He nods until I finally come to my breathless end. "Sounds like a disaster from start to finish." He pauses for effect and then winks. "Luckily, you met me. It just so happens that I'm friends with Penny, his missus. Come with me."

And so he leads me back across the room, back across the glare of the gallery's frank lighting, and waves furiously to Penny Lancaster with his other free hand. They air kiss dramatically and then he fulfills his promise. "Penny, this is Katherine. She is a fabulous writer for the *Telegraph*'s Spy column, and she would love to chat to your other half." Penny looks suspicious for a moment and then appraises me. I guess that she decides that I don't look too scary, because the next thing she does is call across the group, asking Rod to come over and meet someone.

When he sees me, he cracks a wry smile. "You again?" But before I can explain myself or apologize that it is indeed me *again*, Penny jumps in. "Katherine is a writer and she just wants a moment of your time." Then they walk away and Rod is left there, with just me.

"Alright, so you have my attention. What do you want?"

"Um, yes, well, I was just, well, my boss was actually." I cannot form a sentence for the life of me. "Rod, I just want to know your honest op op op opinion of the *X Ffff Factor* contestants?"

"They sent you to ask me that, hoping that I would tell you that they are all utter shit?"

I'm not sure if he means that they sent the "stuttering girl" so he would feel sorry for me and open up. It is hard to tell if he is angry, sarcastic, or just testing me out. I assume it is the latter, "Sure. If that's what you really think, I'm sure they would love me to write that." I decide to throw in some flattery. "Or you ccc c could tell me that the next Rod Stewart is ammmmmmongst them."

It doesn't work. He barely cracks a smile, "Well, I wouldn't take it that far. If you want my opinion, the singers aren't great right now, but some of them have the potential to be pretty decent. You can print that in your paper." With that he extends his hand to shake and begins to move away. His last few words are swallowed by the turn of his shoulder and the swell of the party, but I think I catch them. I think I hear him tell me to get out of the journo industry, that it's the wrong business for a girl like me.

It may have been a reflection of his own tussles with the media, it may have been his take on the cutthroat nature of the industry, or he may have just been commenting on my awkward approach. It is possible that my mind created the words I expected him to say, and he never said anything at all. I'm sure there were a hundred ways to take his warning, but I knew what he was really saying. I *knew* that he was telling me how limited I was as a human being, how there was no way that I could be a stutterer and a journalist.

IT TURNS out that careers are a sticky subject for stutterers. Many advocates argue that any job is possible. They have a point. I have met stutterers in every career that, at twenty-two years old, I had assumed were nigh on impossible. I met stutterers who believed that what they did was far more important than how they said it: journalists, lecturers, doctors, actors, teachers, motivational speakers, pilots, emergency phone operators, and saleswomen who decided to follow what was interesting to them rather than choosing a "safe," quiet career.

I have even met wildly successful speech therapists who stutter.

However, when I made my entrance into the very grown-up workplace, I had only seen posters in speech therapy offices detailing the breadth of careers that stutterers could have. Kindly looking therapists had pointed out Carly Simon, John Stossel, and Jack Welch at every turn. They wanted to prove to me that I could have any job I wanted. Their hearts were in the right place, but there was one rather large problem. They gave me the distinct impression that any job was possible as long as there wasn't a discernible speech impediment. I could have anything I wanted as long as I didn't stutter obviously. Carly, John, and Jack might be stutterers, technically, but they weren't blocking or repeating on every other word.

If you have the advocates on one hand, you have the realists on the other. They appreciate the sentiment that no job is impossible, but they refuse to drink the Kool-Aid. Instead they take to emphasizing the degree of the stutter. What may be possible for a mild stutterer is not always possible for someone who stalls on every word.

Jamie Rocchio is a firecracker of a woman with a master's degree in human development from the University of Rhode Island. She is now retired, and she used to clean houses for a living. "To have continued in the field of psychology, I would have had to keep renewing my license, which wasn't a problem until they made an oral exam mandatory. Put me in a situation like that and I can't speak at all," Jamie explains dynamically through a series of blocks and rapid-fire syllables, "It stopped me from doing what I wanted to do. I think there's a reality about different levels of stuttering. If you can't talk in an oral exam, how can you convince them that when you're in a one-on-one with the client the stuttering doesn't seem to get in the way? You can't."

Is that discrimination? The word is so loaded, so heavy with meaning. It is not a word bandied about too easily. Can a stutterer do any job, can you convince an employer that you are capable of any job? I want to shout out a resounding yes. Yes, we can do any job that we are confident in, we can make it work, we can do anything that we are truly passionate about. And yet I stand firm with the realists on some subjects. On the spectrum of stuttering, I consider myself towards the severe end and, however secure I feel in my abilities, I would never take a job as an emergency call operator, and I would rethink my passion for air traffic control. I would not want a life balancing on the slippery success of my fluency or the speed of my delivery.

In the job market I rarely got to the point where I saw any blatant prejudice, but I heard about it from others. I heard about stutterers who were told not to speak up in work meetings, men who were casually told by their bosses that they would never be promoted as long as they stuttered. In ninth grade, comedy writer Rob Bloom had a guidance counselor who told him that, since he couldn't talk, he "should just become a circus clown." Further along in his academic career, Nick Richard was working on completing his master's in engineering when he was told by a charming faculty member that he "needed to be fluent by graduation or else have the same chance of getting a job as a black guy."

Racism, sexism, ageism. They are all hushed words in the workplace, but the reality is not as pretty as we would like it to be. The truth is that people are looked over because of everything from their weight and their nationality to the color of their skin. As I left the cozy confines of university, I was beginning to realize that adulthood was not as attractive as I had always believed. Having run towards it for years, I quickly tried to start backpedaling.

The transition into the real world is never easy for anyone but it is felt especially painfully for those who stutter. Jim Day is now a human resources and organization development expert at 7-Eleven corporate offices in Dallas, but he grew up as a Mormon in Utah. He explains that "in the church I was cocooned and there was a sense of family." He does not remember any trace of overt stuttering growing up and would never have classified himself as a stutterer. However, at the age of nineteen he was sent to Australia as a missionary for two years and, in his words, "for the first time I could remember, I couldn't talk."

As I graduated from Durham, I walked away from the safety of my friends and the protection of academia into a world for which I felt woefully unprepared. I was afraid that I was doomed. I knew that my stutter wasn't going to hide as quietly as it had before. For the first time in my life it would be a problem for me on a daily basis. In the adult world of earning a living, my stutter was going to get in the way; it was not going to go unnoticed. I was going to be seen by others as disabled, no matter how I saw myself. Jim Day believes that discrimination is rife within the workplace. Having secured his master's and built up a strong résumé, he was laid off after September 11. As he started to look for work, he "got lots of calls that would start off enthusiastically and then, as they heard me stuttering, I would hear the energy of the interview just die. I suspect that they thought I was nervous or had some kind of an intellectual disability."

I had no proof at the time, but I believed that intolerance was lurking everywhere, so I began to ready myself in expectation. I was so vigilantly on the lookout for some frightful discrimination that I recklessly anticipated its advances. I didn't apply for drama clubs and I didn't get involved with the big four company interviewers that prowled our university for candidates. Instead, after graduating I went traveling for a year to escape, to clear my head, and decide what I wanted to do. I interned at an art magazine and at a television station in New York, I worked for a charity in Kenya, and I bummed around Southeast Asia, all under the guise of discovering myself, of searching for whatever my dream job might be. I loved the adventure, excitement, and novelty of it all, but I didn't find my calling. In all honesty, I had always known what I wanted to be.

Since I was a child I had always dreamed of being a writer. I had no idea how I would make a living, but for years I had pictured myself in a romantic cottage in France where I would write my novels on vintage typewriters and hold fabulous soirées with my friends. Durham had solidified those dreams. Writing my final history dissertation on the Vietnam War, I had lived for a month in Boston's JFK library. I had worn out my highlighters and come home carrying boxes of government files. I had relished the excitement of organizing my notes, of pulling together my research, and forming my thesis. Writing my dissertation, I had learnt about the stuttering war correspondent Homer Bigart, and his work had inspired me to temporarily forgo the fictional French idyll and earn a living as a journalist.

And yet, when I finally returned to London, I stayed up at night worrying that the dreams that my parents had for me, the dreams that I had for myself, might never come true. I had no idea how anyone carved out a career as a writer, but I assumed that becoming a journalist was a good gateway. And yet, as I started going to interviews, working part-time jobs, and applying for fancy internships, I worried that my stutter would stop me from getting a job that I loved. I worried about the simple question of how I was going to earn a living when I couldn't even get a job as a receptionist answering the telephone. As I walked in and out of recruiters' offices, I knew that somehow I was going to have to find a way to earn money, to carve out a career, and to prove that I was worthy of respect, that I was more than just a "stutterer."

When an editor at a newspaper internship pulled me aside to tell me that I needed to do one thing to advance my journalism career, I was already armed and ready with a counterattack. When she told me that I should take typing classes, that typing articles with two fingers was not the speediest option out there, I was struck mute. I had been readying myself to tell her that I would advance with my stutter in tow, that I did not need to be fluent to succeed, that it would not hold me back. My now defunct comeback sat heavily on my tongue and paralyzed me.

Looking back over those years of job hunting, I know that I always worried more about my speech than others ever did, that I was the only person who ever truly held myself back. No one else was closing doors on me, I was closing them myself as I tried to search for safety. Everything looks far less catastrophic in hindsight, but when I was trying to find work as a journalist, I did everything in my power to hide my stutter. In the newsroom I pretended that I was simply a quiet and focused worker. I rarely spoke up in meetings, dodged any whiff of a conference call, and walked miles around London rather than call up a story lead with a question. The process was exhausting, and I knew that I would never be a truly great journalist. Eventually, I couldn't handle the daily fear, and I convinced myself that it was better to go into a job that was less combative, less centered on talking. Something more research based. I started looking into all my friends' jobs in sensible occupations like banking, accountancy, and law. I told myself that it was about the money, that I needed to ditch the ridiculous dream of writing and get a job that would actually help me pay the rent.

I had lots of good, sensible reasons for moving into asset management. None of them had anything to do with stuttering. The pendulum shift surprised everyone, but it seemed sensible enough, reasonable enough. So no one asked any questions when I took up a job as an in-house investment writer. I carried on denying the fact that my stutter was starting to rule my life. I kept that up for well over a year.

Then it all came tumbling down.

• • •

IN SOME distant office the phone rings once. I contemplate hanging up before I take this charade any further.

Then I remember caller ID and suspect he will call me back if I hang up. Instead, I subconsciously hold my breath and look down at my briefly scribbled notes. Unsuccessfully, I try to release the air caught in my throat.

The man, we'll call him Charles, works at a rating agency. He is compiling the latest report of one of our struggling funds, and after a meeting with the fund manger last week, I have been answering his various follow-up questions in emails. When he called an hour ago, I had heard my phone ringing and had hidden by the printer, pretending not to notice, until it stopped. For the past fifty-nine minutes I have been psyching myself up to call him back. I had considered emailing, but I expected that he would just call again and I needed to give the impression that we are confident, meticulous, and organized. That the small blip in the fund's performance is nothing to worry about.

The phone rings again.

I pass the seconds by conjuring an image of the genius that designed our open-plan office and picture myself sticking pins in him. My heart races in my aching chest. I question my sanity.

Silently, I beg for the call to go to voicemail. Then he picks up. "Charles speaking."

His voice screams of a British boarding school education. My sane thoughts are bullied into submission. I picture him leaning back in his chair, his recently polished leather shoes resting cockily on the desk in front of him. It is far more likely that he is sitting in some cramped cubicle with no windows, but I can't help but imagine him taking in the view from his corner office overlooking Canary Wharf.

I am on the verge of a panic attack and, as I clutch the phone to my ear, I realize that anxiety has locked my voice, trapped it into silence.

"Hello? Is there anyone there?"

I have to say something, I have to get past the point of him thinking I am a disturbed prank caller. I beg my voice to come out. My mouth gapes open in the familiar tongue gagging shape of a *K*. Worried that he will hang up any second, I push out one long convoluted sound. "This is Kaaaaaaaaaaa Kaaaaaaa." I have expelled something, but now the secret is out. Either he knows I stutter or he thinks that I am having some sort of epileptic fit. Neither fills me with joy.

"Hello, who is this?"

The man has a talent for sounding simultaneously confused and bored. I rein in my charging emotions. I tell myself that I only have eight more letters to get through. "J J J J J JJJJJ just give me a second here. This is K K K K K KK."

I begin making the shapes of each individual letter with my finger on the desk. It's a desperate action that I haven't done in years, and I have no idea why I think it will help me. I just want to trick my brain into letting the word come free: "Kaaaaa Kaaa t t therine."

"I didn't catch that, could you repeat yourself?"

Having barely made it through the first time, I have no desire to relive the experience. My words are hanging limply in the space between us. I picture Charles looking impatiently at his watch.

Subconsciously my eyes roll downwards in defeat, and I stare at my keyboard. In my peripheral vision I can see my coworkers. In our now silent office, they have all suddenly found their monthly fund prospectuses and are staring at them with unusual fascination. I suspect that they are trying to be kind, not to catch my eye, but all I can sense is their pity. My stutter has locked us all in this communal humiliation. The shame makes me frantic.

"Hi, this is K K K K K." I shut my eyes tight and then flick them open, an old trick that looks bizarre but sometimes works to propel out a word. I kick myself for doing it. "Hi, this is K K K K Kaaa Kaaatherine Preston."

I feel like I have broken some bad news to him. I can hear a slight sigh from the other side of the line. Then, before I can explain why I am calling, he regains his cocky, schoolboy swagger and pipes up. "Did you just forget your name?"

To add insult to injury, he concludes his hilarious witticism with a rolling laugh. As thoughtless as he sounds, I honestly doubt that he has any idea that I stutter. And yet, whatever his reasoning, his words catalyze my mounting anxiety and turn it into fierce anger. Does he think this is some private joke I play on everyone? Is stuttering really so unusual? Is it more likely that he has managed to speak to someone so incredibly stupid or with such debilitating amnesia?

Emotion clogs my voice and cracks my composure. My body has leapt free of my control. The silence drags on the line. With my heart pounding I panic.

Still holding the phone to my ear, I surreptitiously pull out the cord. The call immediately disconnects, but I sit there still pretending to listen. I throw in some "ums" and "ahs" for effect. And then I execute a dramatic mood shift. "Hello? I can't hear you anymore. Hello?" I frown and look puzzled. I worry that I may be overacting just a tad.

Finally, I conclude my performance and replace the phone into its cradle. Then I plaster a smile on my face and look up at my coworkers, "Must have lost him, he was on his mobile, bad reception."

I stand up from my desk and, with as much poise as I can muster, totter to the women's bathroom. I walk in and scan the stalls for any telltale shoes. Having verified that I'm alone, I clutch the cold marble of the sink and face myself in the mirror. I look at my eyeliner and mascara, at my suit and my high heels. I close my eyes in disgust. I remember the interview when I first applied for the job. How cocky I had been telling my employers that my stutter wasn't an issue for me, that it shouldn't be an issue for them.

Here I am, more than a year later, hanging up on clients and pathetically hiding in the bathroom.

Tears begin to pool in my closed eyes and I force myself to open them. I watch the tears fall down my face. I take in my shaking hands and study the swelled redness of my cheeks. What an impostor.

I have spent my life saying that my stutter doesn't bother me. I have kept it a dirty secret. It is not that I'm reticent about the fact I stutter; it was never something I could hide. However, my answers had never veered into any realm that could lead to pity. I am ever the optimist.

"No, my stutter's not a big deal."

"No, I don't see it as a disability."

"Yes, I have stuttered for most of my life."

"No, it has never held me back."

It is a script that I know well. It feeds neatly into the image I want to have of myself, the image I want others to see. I'm tough, I can handle anything, I'm strong, I never feel sorry for myself.

Suddenly that all seems like utter rubbish. I am petrified, overwhelmed, exhausted, and not at all courageous. In fact, looking at the pathetic figure I cut in the mirror I realize how deeply ashamed and scared I feel.

I torture myself by picturing how I must have looked when I was speaking down the telephone. I have seen myself speaking in videos and am well aware of the way I appear. My mouth shudders viciously. I clench and throw open my eyes in desperation. Sometimes my shoulders or my head flick and jerk. Cruelly, I play back the guttural grunt that I made as I pushed out the first letter of my name.

I have always thought of raw, unbridled emotions as being the privilege of others. I don't like to complain, I don't enjoy talking about my problems, and I certainly don't lose control of my sanity in the office bathroom.

And yet here I am. The tears are starting to fall more heavily and I am beginning to gasp for breath. I rush into one of the stalls to escape the potential embarrassment of anyone else seeing me in such a state of abandon. The now flooding tears shake my body and make me clutch at the sides of the stall for support.

I hear the bathroom door open, so I pick up my legs and

crouch on the toilet. I hold my breath and swallow the gasps as I wait for whoever it is to leave. When I know I am alone again, I whisper my name fluently amidst my hiccupping breaths. I desperately need to hear the sound of my own voice, and, alone, I know I will not stutter. It is reassuring and melancholic to hear the fluid syllables flow from my mouth.

"What is going to happen to me?"

What happens to someone who loves to talk, someone who hates silence, and someone who has continued to stutter well into adulthood? I'm finding out. Perched on a toilet, talking to myself on the sixth floor of a London office building. It is not pretty, but I can see the dust settling, I can see what I want.

I want to sound like everyone else. I don't want to worry about picking up the phone. I don't want to be scared of meeting strangers. I don't want to feel handicapped and weak. I want to be witty and eloquent. I want to be fluent.

I need a cure.

CHAPTER 7

MISSION FOR A CURE

Henley, February 2008

THINK THAT I know what speech therapists are meant to look like. In my mind they are limp-wristed, soft-spoken women who are barely out of puberty and barely strong enough to carry their weighty promises of fluency. They are not meant to be manicured, formidable creatures with strong opinions and easy laughs. Anne defies my expectations.

I had first met the woman who would change my life when I was sixteen. It was the year that university interviews started to loom, the year that I realized my success rested on something less tangible than getting good grades. I knew that if I was going to be accepted at a great university, I was going to need to impress them with my verbal aptitude.

I suspect it was pretty obvious how much the thought petrified me. My mum had seen a documentary showing a new three-day speech therapy course called the Starfish program. They had talked about "costal breathing," something she had never heard of, and the show had depicted one boy's journey before, during, and after the life-altering course. Mum had been impressed enough by the program director, Anne, to brave the subject one evening. After years of angrily silencing her whenever she brought up the subject, I bit my lip and nodded. I told her that it sounded alright, that I wouldn't mind giving them I call.

However nonchalant I wanted to come across, I had gone on her intensive course full of hope, praying that it would work. It did help, for a short time. I was the only kid on the course and it was the first time I had met adult stutterers, the first time I had mentors in my life who knew what it was like. I watched in awe as deliberate and fluent words came spilling out of their mouths. It was easy to be fluent with them on the course, but in the aftermath it all got a bit more tricky. I couldn't bring myself to use the new speaking techniques that she taught me. I was still desperate to fit in, and talking in a voice akin to Darth Vader's did not look like the ticket to winning any popularity contests. So I didn't change, not in the end, and I believed, yet again, that it was my fault. I believed that I didn't work hard enough, that I hadn't wanted it badly enough.

However, by the age of twenty-three, I am desperate again. I suspect that Anne is my best bet. She is the most determined and passionate speech therapist I know. I'm ready to follow her blindly.

A deep red blush pricks at my cheeks as I pick up the phone. It is like calling up an ex-boyfriend whom I've heartlessly dumped and then wantonly ignored for seven years. I fully expect her to hang up on me, but I have no choice. If I don't call I'm quite likely to lose my job as well as my sanity.

"Hi Aaaaa aaa aaaa aaa . . ." I take another shallow breath, "A a a a a aaaaaa aaaaa a . . ."

I can't get it out. I start crying. What a disappointment. I pull the receiver away from my ear and grip the solid wood of the kitchen table. I consider hanging up. The whole situation is too pathetic. I am not sure that I can get out my name at all. I fear that I may stand here forever saying one letter into the silence of the line. I take a deep breath and carry on. Because what options do I have? I'm afraid of what will happen if I don't try.

"Hi, Aa a a a anne. It is K k k k ka ka ka ka kath kath kath Katherine."

"Katherine. How lovely to hear from you."

Nothing. No recriminations. No reaction to my stutter. She remembers me. Or at least I assume she does. I'm so used to being made memorable by my stutter that it doesn't dawn on me that she must get constant calls from people who sound just like me, that I'm not all that unusual to her. Only later do I wonder if she recognized me or if she reacts the same way to every stutterer who calls.

At the time I breathe an audible sigh of relief. I am still crying but more quietly now; it has turned into a sniffling version of its former self. My words make their way forward, shakily intact: "Aaa anne, I want to come back."

"How soon?" She hasn't heard from me since the previous millennium, but she doesn't miss a beat.

"As soon as you'll have me." I catch a glimpse of my puffy face in the kitchen mirror. Needy is not a good look. "Or you you you you know, whenever the n n n n n next available course is. I kn kn kno kno know that you get bbbbb bbbbb b bbb booked up about a year in advance."

"Our next course is in two weeks. I would love you to come. I'll make room for you."

A smile slips across my mouth, and relief unclenches my fisted fingers and toes. I am like a dripping tap. Having been able to count the number of times I have cried on one hand for most of my life, I can't stop the flood anymore. "Th th th th thank you."

"Don't thank me. You are welcome back on any course at any time. But Katherine." She pauses heavily. "Don't come for me. Come for you. You will be coming as a refresher, so you'll be teaching the technique to the new people. Can you do that? Can you make this work for you?" She pauses for a few more long seconds. "It's been a long time."

I can hear that she wants me to come back, but I feel her disappointment sharply. I am sure it was lack of hard work that held me back before and am convinced that this time will be different. This time I am more determined. "I c c c c can. I'll see you in two weeks. Thank you, Anne."

As I hang up I imagine what it would be like to be an alcoholic who has finally joined AA or a manic depressive who has chosen to see a psychiatrist. I feel a strange kinship with those who are broken, those who want to be fixed, those who are desperate. My surrender makes me childlike, and I'm scared. It is lucky that I turn to Anne. Had the Moonies happened to call, I'm certain that I would have signed away my life on the dotted line. I want a savior.

Two weeks later I rattle in my chair as we drive to the south coast. I shake for all that Anne might tell me, for all the ways I will need to change to rid myself of my stutter. I shake at the thought of no longer being the "stutterer" I have always been. For once I can think of no small talk to ease the enormity of the situation, I can't joke it off anymore. Feverishly I swing from regret to hopefulness.

The course is being held in a barn behind a countryside hotel. My mum has come with me; I have asked her there to say thank you for all the other times she tried to help, all the times that I screamed at her for bringing up speech therapy as I was growing up. I have asked her to join me because I need her to be there. I need a witness. I'm not sure that I'm strong enough on my own. She slips into the conference room behind me and urges me forward. I may have a career, my own flat, and my own car, but I am regressing quickly back to adolescence. Hard brown-cushioned seats are arranged in ten neat lines. I barely take in the room as I beeline towards a seat a few rows from the front.

Five groups are clustered around the edge of the room and a few other loners are sitting by themselves. I don't recognize any faces. I watch as more people wander in. Middle-aged men, punk rocker girls, elderly women, and couples. A guy who looks like he is a few years older than me comes to sit next to me. Embarrassed, I pretend to look for something in my bag. He introduces himself using the deep-breathing technique that I remember. He explains that he is a refresher coming back to help the newbies. I nod and congratulate him. Anne walks in, and her entrance saves me from having to out myself as a refresher as well. All eyes turn to her as she waves at friends, hugs people, squeezes shoulders, laughs at the end of some jokes, and makes her way towards the front of the room.

"Will all the first timers come and sit in the first row?" I recognize her warm, no-nonsense way of speaking, her immaculate hair, her power suit. Suddenly I'm grateful that she asked me back as a refresher. Because I can see beyond the shifting bodies, I remember what the first timers have to do. I can see the shape of the video camera and a lone seat opposite. I watch the first timers shift tentatively forward to take their seats. They never lose sight of the menacing machine.

"Welcome all of you to the Starfish program." She impresses me just as she always did. Fluent as she is, she speaks using the technique. Breathy, deep tone, sharp inhalation, chest forward, project your voice, "I'm Anne Blight, and there is so much that I want to talk to you about. However, there's no point in me saying much right now because I know that none of you will hear much of it, I know what you're all looking at." She smiles knowingly. It is not her first rodeo. There are a few nervous sniggers from the front and a couple of laughs from the refreshers in the back. We are all in on the joke. We know how much we hate watching ourselves speak, how much we hate having our utterances recorded. We are all scared of seeing ourselves played back at some future date. She explains that all first timers will be asked to take the seat opposite the camera, to make their "before" videos. She asks for the first volunteer.

I can feel the lurch in their collective stomach. An older man shudders towards the seat. As the recording starts, his stuttered speech is slurred and difficult to understand. Anne asks him a few questions and then he is given a passage to read out loud. He often looks to the floor, looks pleadingly at Anne, fitfully flicks his head backwards but carries on.

At the end of the ordeal, he is enthusiastically clapped and cheered back to the row of first timers. He smiles thankfully. He looks exhausted. I exhale, feeling nauseous. I realize I have been holding my breath through most of his speech.

Once all the first timers have made their videos Anne pulls back our attention by bellowing, "I hope you haven't come here for two things. I hope that you haven't come here for a cure, and I hope that you haven't come here for fluency. Because we don't have either of those. There is no cure! And anyone who claims to have one is wrong." Her words quickly crush my misguided hopes and replace them with new anticipation. "You don't have a disease. You have a habit, and we can change habits." The idea of stuttering as a habit bothers me, but I can't find an adequate reason why. It just seems wrong to equate something as pervasive as stuttering to fingernail biting. The unformed thought is drowned out by Anne's thundering words. Emotion thickens her voice as she crescendos, "But you *can* have faith in this technique."

I recognize one of the men who moves forward to teach us all the first baby steps. He was on my first course. A big, burly, and vulnerable retired truck driver. Not easily forgettable. He has a cloth belt straining slightly around his wide chest. He explains that we are changing the way we speak. The technique has a respectable lineage. Politicians and opera singers use it, and apparently Lionel Logue used it to treat King George VI. It is based on something called costal breathing and it is all about timing. A sharp inhale, a few deeply spoken words, and then an exhale of all the remaining air.

The cloth belts are unusual. I have never seen them used in any other therapy. The belts sit tightly around our chests so we can feel that we are taking the "right" breath. We wear them over our shirts and T-shirts, and they make us look like some kind of strange army ready to go to war against our stutters. They look strangest on the women, who fiddle with the Velcro and laugh as their breasts are pushed unattractively downwards and a slight bulge appears under their armpits. Those who complain are reproached and encouraged to feel proud of wearing something that is helping them. They are reminded that there is no shame in everyone knowing that they are working on their speech.

Wearing the belt makes the whole process more physical, makes it easier to know what should feel right when everything feels strange. A "proper" deep and quick breath makes the belt cinch tightly around our flesh. If you can't feel the belt straining against your chest, you aren't doing it right. In theory it sounds like the easiest thing in the world. I know that it's not, but I push away my cynicism. I want to be swept away, I want to be one of the faithful.

We rearrange the seats to face each other in pairs snaking

around the room. As a "refresher," I am assigned as a teacher to a new student. At first I pity the poor sod who gets me, but I'm grateful to have a reason to start talking to someone and surprised to feel how quickly the technique comes back to me. Speaking in the safety of the conference room is easy, luxuriously easy. It always has been. The familiar surroundings seem to ignite some latent memory, and I start to enjoy teaching the technique, feeling the strong, deep voice bubbling up from my diaphragm. I enjoy seeing my student's transformation, watching the shocked relief on his face the first time he says his name fluidly.

I start to feel light-headed; all the deep breathing, the communal ecstasy of the room, is getting to me. My English sarcasm is being tested beyond its natural limits, and I'm becoming a sentimental mess watching everyone. There may as well be a *Gladiator* soundtrack playing behind me.

For the three days of the course, from sunrise until we prop up the hotel bar at midnight, we support each other, we smile in encouragement, and we call each other out for not using the technique. Any skepticism is squashed by the ridiculous joy of simply saying my name fluently, of calling up the hotel reception, of telling someone where I live. The feeling is addictive. Towards the end of the course, I lose all my reserve and stand up and tell everyone that I'm a "proud recovering stutterer." I see my mum grinning at me and looking tearily around the room.

I walk out of the course cockily fluent. I call up directory inquiries ten times on the drive home. Mum and I giggle like schoolkids. I can't wait to see my dad and show off my "new voice" to my friends. No one can stop me. I'll call up other attendees from the course every night after work. I will wear my cloth belt every day. When I'm feeling brave I'll wear it over my jumper. I want people to see it, to ask me about it. I want any excuse to tell people that I'm a "recovering stammerer," no longer one of the pod people.

DR. SCOTT Yaruss, an associate professor at the University of Pittsburgh and director of the Stuttering Center of Western Pennsylvania, has a theory on speech therapy. He believes that "Change only happens when the pain of staying the same is greater than the pain of change." He's right. The difficulties of change are certainly easier to face, to embrace, when we are exhausted by the difficulties of our current reality. And yet, even when you are desperate for change, even when you are ready to cling onto any lifeline that comes your way, even when you are prepared to put your faith in a technique, changing your speech is never easy.

In the wake of the three-day course, I called up other attendees every night. I wore my belt and breathed heavily down the phone as I heard about their challenges, their families, and their journey back into domesticity. I got dressed for work and almost walked out of my house with the belt strapped cockily over my shirt. But I couldn't get past my front door. I compromised and wore it under my shirt, but my skin was hot, raw, and chafed at the end of the day. Looking at the small red welts under my armpits I told myself that I should take it off, that it was hurting me. I couldn't admit to myself that I was

ashamed of wearing it in public, yet I refused even to enter-
tain the thought of wearing it over my clothes. I compromised
with my warring conscience. I would carry the belt around in
my handbag. If I needed it for a meeting, I would quickly run
in the bathroom and put it on.

I carried on trying to change the way I spoke without the
belt's constraint. I practiced my breathing techniques every
morning in the shower and on the way to the Underground.
I spoke three words per breath, I paused, I stopped myself
from taking any "top-up breaths." The problem was that now
I really was talking funny. I had replaced one strange way of
speaking with a voice that made every sentence into a procla-
mation, that didn't allow for a spontaneous aside, that didn't
incorporate any tonal or rhythmic variation. I sounded me-
chanical, soulless. I didn't sound like myself.

I shared my worries with some of the more devoted followers of the course, those who had been using the technique
for years. Their responses generally fell into four categories.

"You have to use the technique all day every day. That is
the only way to get rid of your stutter."

"Would you rather have fluency or fast, 'natural' speech?"

"This is how politicians talk; you should be proud of
sounding so authoritative."

"You are the only one that thinks you sound strange."

I wasn't so sure. I saw the way people reacted. I saw their
bored expressions as my new condescendingly slow voice
maimed the pace of every conversation. All my friends had
grown accustomed to my stutter, and they were ill-prepared
for my new strangeness.

In fairness, no one ever voiced any of my worries, but I still saw their reactions, or I thought I did. I stumbled on "proof" years later when I spoke to Nick Richard, a graduate of a very similar therapy called the McGuire Program. Nick explained how an old friend of his had articulated all of my concerns, "I had just been to a refresher day so my voice was very strong, deep, loud, and my friend was very thrown off by it," he remembered. "I tried to explain to her why I have to do this and why it's important to do it all the time. She said, 'You don't stutter with me anyway, so can't you just do it when you need to do it.' I tried to explain that it's not about fluency per se but about being disciplined and consistent, and she replied, 'Well, I don't really like the way that you talk now, so could you just go back to speaking the way you talked before.'"

Nick's friend is probably the exception. But she voiced all of the worries that I harbored at the time. At the heart of it all I believed that I was no longer a good communicator. My chat was forced, my banter boring. I could say anything I wanted, but I couldn't enjoy saying it. I may have been technically fluent, but I sounded like one of my distant relatives who spoke in such a slow drone that we fought over who would answer the phone when he called.

Perhaps the deliberate, monotone voice of the "costal breather" was annoying to no one but myself. I will never know because, having left the course confident, I started to feel self-conscious and ashamed in my real life. I modified my technique. I went against Anne's recommendation. I used my "natural" voice when I was with friends and started using the technique only when I thought I might stutter, when I really needed it. I tried to bring it into action when I was on the phone or when I was speaking to strangers, but I found that when I needed it the most, when I desperately wanted to be fluent, it didn't work. I started questioning everything, so I went back to the course. I had my three-day fix and returned to work with renewed conviction. The vicious cycle continued. I couldn't make myself feel good about using my new voice in public, and I couldn't bring the techniques to the forefront when I most needed them. I grappled with the challenge of focusing on using the speaking techniques while actually saying something worthwhile. The joy of conversation was decimated.

I have been told by some stutterers who have "succeeded" that I was lazy, that I didn't work at it hard enough. Stutterers are not always the supportive, united front you may expect. We can be our own harshest critics. We even have our own polarized gangs; imagine the Sharks and the Jets but with a lot less dancing and a lot more strongly worded letters.

When I first learnt about the different therapy approaches, it seemed as if there were two distinct schools of thought. One school believed that the goal of therapy should be 100 percent fluency, that stuttering should be treated as a purely physical condition. They believed that you had to succumb entirely to a new speaking technique, that you had to retrain your speech and relearn how to talk. They insisted that you had to wave good-bye to your old voice and usher in a new persona. Many of them believed that therapy could be successful for anyone, that it just took determination and rigor-ous hard work. Some promised a quick fix, others maintained that speech therapy was a long and difficult process. They had a toolbox of jargon-heavy approaches at their disposal. I interviewed therapists who taught everything from pausing to the unfortunately named chunking, easy onset, metronomic speech, and stretched continuous vowels.

Many of the therapists experimented with different approaches and tried to tailor their program to each individual patient. Other therapists offered a one-size-fits-all approach that aimed to mold each student to a "proven" treatment. Many of the adherents to these singular "fluency shaping" programs believed that their journey could be translated universally. Blind jazz guitarist Eric Warren graduated from one such program, the Hollins Communications Research Institute. To all appearances, he no longer has any discernible speech impediment. In his words, "I have proven that, if you go through these physical techniques, you will not stutter."

Founded in 1972 by Dr. Ronald L. Webster, the Hollins Institute quickly became infamous in the stuttering world. It is adored by those who found "success" there (those who now see themselves as fluent) and hated by those who feel tricked by their high claims of fluency. The program's clinicians claim to have treated approximately six thousand clients in the forty years they have been in existence. Their treatment is based on a target approach where students are taught to make the "right" sounds. The program is regimented, focused on saying a certain number of syllables per breath, changing the way patients breathe, and contouring their sounds to fit a specific form. If the students make the "wrong" sound, a red light flashes. The process carries on for twelve days in the confines of the treatment center. At the end of the course, students are expected to take their "new voice" into the outside world. It is a stark, black-and-white world of good and bad where every stuttered word is an act of failure and any student's inability to gain fluency is his own fault.

If the "fluency shapers" are aiming to eradicate the stutter by changing the way we speak, another school of speech therapy wants to change the way we stutter. Pioneered by stutterer and researcher Charles Van Riper, the so-called "stuttering modifiers" focus on the moments of stuttering in order to improve communication but not necessarily increase fluency. Their goal is to teach their patients to stutter in a different way, a better way, to create a relaxed and fluid form of stuttering. Van Riper taught his followers to use techniques such as light contact, pull-outs, and cancellations to change the experience of speech before, during, and after a stutter. Both fluency shaping and stuttering modification have their adherents and their critics, and neither eclipses the other in terms of success.

Having assumed that stuttering therapy was a monochrome world of only two schools of thought, I was surprised to see that many modern therapists were rejecting the outdated notions of labels and boxes and were starting to merge the two. These therapists believe that each stutterer is different, that each person has a unique reaction and has to forge his or her own path. They have thrown away their soapboxes and are no longer preaching. They are fans of the "whatever works" school of speech therapy. They steer clear of the tempting trap to blame their client if the speech therapy does not help. Instead, they take their cues from talk therapy. They believe in counseling, in listening, and in teaching self-acceptance along with presenting a toolkit of speaking techniques. They focus on the psychological compensations that fall in the stutter's wake and consider all the ways that nervousness and shame can exacerbate the disorder. They try to find a technique that is better suited to their client's specific needs.

Today I tend to lean towards the middle ground, towards therapists like the portrayal of Lionel Logue in *The King's Speech*. I'm attracted to those magnetic people who focus on building a relationship above adhering to a specific doctrine. I no longer believe I failed because I couldn't make a technique work for me. Instead, I believe that we need a better understanding. Stuttering is a condition with far more questions than answers. We still do not know exactly why stuttering occurs, and thus every attempt at speech therapy is an exercise in trial and error. Perhaps the label "stutterer" is unhelpful in itself. Are we all the same? Probably not. Maybe stuttering encompasses a slew of differing conditions.

Whatever the answer, it is clear that there is no one obvious path. No therapy approach should claim to work for everyone; no therapist should claim to have the definitive answer. There is no one right way and no unanimously agreed-upon approach to treatment. Fluency is not the product of straightforward hard work. Practice does not always make perfect.

Sadly, I learnt all of this later. In my midtwenties I was still searching for answers. I wanted a magic cure, and yet the treatment that I had found was making me miserable, inhibiting my emotions, and stifling my conversations. I was just as drained and exhausted as I had been before therapy. The only reason I carried on was because I loved the other characters I had met in the course. I didn't want to let them down, I didn't want to let Anne down. So I carried on calling them most nights. I heard about Graham's home renovation, about Guy's family, about Marek's work with schoolchildren. I loved hearing their voices, I loved that I was becoming part of a supportive world where everyone understood each other's deepest vulnerabilities.

"WHY DON'T you tell your colleagues that you're using a new speaking technique?"

It is early autumn and I have just finished my second Starfish course. I'm high on fluency but nervous about going back to the office again. Despite the fact that my long-suffering HR department has paid for both of my courses, I have not told any of my colleagues where I have been for the weekend. I have called up Guy to whine, and he is coming up with advice that is far too sensible.

"If you're worried about their reactions to your new speech, why don't you just tell them what's happening and how you would like them to react? Problem solved."

He's a lovely, kind chap, and he has a fair point. So I sit down to type the email the next morning. I will just send it out to a select few. I'll keep it all very factual. I don't want a pity party. I'll just tell them that I've been on a course, that I'm using a deep-breathing technique (in case they worry that I'm perpetually hyperventilating), and that I'd appreciate if they looked me in the eye, if they didn't rush me, if they gave me a few extra seconds to speak my words slowly and deliberately.

Rather than type in everyone's emails individually I decide to do a mass email to the company and selectively erase the email addresses of those that I don't fancy baring my soul to. Asset management is not the most touchy-feely of industries. Sending it to everyone feels akin to the nightmarish scenario of walking into the office naked.

So I start erasing emails. I start with the top floor, calmly erasing the names of the fund managers. I move down a floor, then the clock ticks to 8:45 A.M. and my colleagues start arriving. I keep hiding the email and then opening it again when no one is looking. My boss sits down next to me. I pretend to be looking at the news. Then I open it again to erase a couple more names. And then I press Send.

In hindsight I will remember it as one of those comically buffoonish moments, but at the time I'm struck dumb by my stupidity. Somehow in my desperate flicking between screens I slipped up. Mortally. Frantically I try to reverse the mistake. I can't. I have just sent my Oprah-worthy email to more than a hundred people at our office, most of whom I've barely exchanged a "how do you do" with. I do the only sensible thing. I power walk to the bathroom.

I have spent too much time in the marbled room recently.

I'm annoyed at myself for resorting to my former hiding place. So I give myself a silent pep talk and walk out.

"Katherine, I saw the email. Good luck! You're sounding great."

"Hey, looking forward to hearing this new voice of yours."

"It's really cool that you are working on your speech."

So far it is not too horrendous. Most of the people who have read the email give me a thumbs up as I walk back to my desk. A select few openly stare at me. Fair play. I would stare at me, too.

I open my inbox to a slew of congratulations. Most of them are from people I know, but there are a few people I've never spoken to. "My brother is an alcoholic. He really struggles with it. I've forwarded on your email to give him a boost in the right direction." The comparison is not what I expected, but I write back a heartfelt good luck. It is the least I can do. "I have diabetes and I've always been so ashamed of it. Thanks for making me feel better." My inbox is turning into a confessional booth. I feel like I should be doling out a ten-step process.

For the rest of the day people stop me in the corridors to tell me of their struggles with everything from drugs to diabetes and divorce. My desk starts to resemble a continuous AA meeting. I feel like we have all come out of the closet wearing feather boas and singing show tunes. It is liberating.

But there is one niggling doubt. One question that keeps popping up in my inbox and keeps following me around the spaces of our office, one question that I don't have much of a reply to: "Why do people stutter?" In my mumbling silence, I expect that they are coming up with their own explanations, their own breakdown of my psyche. Maybe they are wondering if I was traumatized as a child, if I had some strange illness, if I am perpetually nervous or hiding some deep, dark secret.

I know that none of those answers are right, and yet I don't know what the truth is. Years ago my parents had let go of the notion that my stutter was caused by my grandma's death, but we had never explored it any further. We had always focused on fixing it. We had always been too focused on the what to dwell too much on the why.

I have no idea what causes stuttering, and I have no idea why the technique is really supposed to work. We are told not to question why it helps, just to believe in it. Yet I realize that the technique is not enough, that I need an explanation, a reason why I stutter and why the technique it supposed to help me. I realize that I need to learn more about my own condition. It embarrasses me that I haven't questioned anything, that I haven't wanted to find out more about the genesis of stuttering.

Later, in the privacy of my little South London pad, I sit on my bed and type "stutter" into Google, and a million quick fixes litter my search results. I type in "stuttering research" and a few more interesting results come up. The first results I see are all in America. The deeper I go into the searches, the more often I see researchers and therapists in Maryland, California, and Illinois pop up on my screen. There is something called the Lidcombe Project, based in Australia, that works solely with children and sounds vaguely similar to the treatment I received years earlier at the Michael Palin Centre, but my initial research uncovers precious little in England. I wonder if financial resources are scarce for a condition that is not life-threatening.

I call up Cat, my best friend from Durham. I start by telling her about the emotional gymnastics of my day. I need to temper the insanity of my decision, to ease her into it slowly. As I run up to the sentence, I can already picture her fiancé rolling his eyes as she tells him later.

"I've decided, I'm going to hand in my resignation."

I have rarely heard her lost for words. The silent seconds are making my throat constrict so I start talking again, "There's more. Or there's a better plan at least. I'm, I'm, I'm, I'm well. I have this idea to move to America to write a book."

There's a relief and a madness in saying it out loud. I have not been happy for a while. My relationship has been limping forward for months in a series of heartwrenching breakups, and makeups and I have been spending my days counting off the hours until my next holiday, or my next happy hour. I have been self-destructively restless for a while, but neither of us thought that I would take it this far. A few weeks ago we were at a friend's wedding in Kenya and I was telling her that I needed to change my life. On holiday it had seemed easy, the best idea in the world. I can't believe that I'm actually thinking of going ahead with it.

"Petit! You're actually going to do this? What are you going to write about?"

She's my closest friend, but we have rarely spoken about my stutter. Oddly, I feel awkward bringing it up now. I start talking about a friend whose biography I'd love to write. I sound halfhearted saying it, though. I can hear myself waffling. I decide to bite the bullet. "There's this other idea. What if I wrote a book on stuttering? On why it happens and who it happens to, on what it means to speak differently."

I don't let her say anything as I gallop onwards. I form the idea as I speak and preempt the questions I think she might ask. "I know that I could just write a few articles, get back into journalism with a few pieces on stuttering. I know that would be the sensible option. But I don't want to be sensible. I want to be daunted by a project that feels unmanageable and exciting, something that has the potential to change things. I want to write a book. And stuttering is the perfect subject; it is the one subject I'm certain I can write about."

My monologue comes to a breathy end, and I remember how we always joked about the novels we would write as we studied for exams in Durham. Cat had a pseudonym all mapped out and a book of stories already entertaining her rowing team. Yet she had graduated to become a management consultant and thrived working in an office. We had always been so similar until we started working. I love how she has it all together, how I can show off my incredibly impressive friend. The house, the chap she always loved, the great job, none of it had been easy to get, but it is obvious how much it all suits her. I wish I could match her contentment. I wish I didn't feel so trapped.

A couple of days ago I was telling her that they had offered me a promotion at work. My boss had just resigned and the space had opened up. I should have been celebrating my climb up the corporate ladder rather than fleeing from it.

"How will you go about it?" Her voice cuts down the line, the no-nonsense tone I imagine she normally reserves for office politics.

"So I have this idea of interviewing as many stutterers, researchers, and sp sp speech therapists as I can and then turning it into a book of oral histories or a journalistic investigation. It makes sense to do all the exploring in America because it seems like they are at the foreffffront of re re re re re." As the stutter lingers on I know that it is not just about the research. That comes into it, but it is really about going to a country where I have no preconceptions, somewhere that I can make a fresh start. I run up at the sentence again: "It seems like America is at the forefront of research, and in England I have too many ideas about therapy and about p p p people. I need to see it all through new eyes."

I'm ready for the pause this time. I'm already planning what I can say to convince her that it makes sense, that I'm not throwing my life away on the whim of some mad idea. But her warm voice comes giggling down the receiver too quickly for me to begin again, "Petit, this is amazing. Completely insane, mind you, but amazing."

Somehow her laughter calms me, I smile for the first time since I picked up the phone. Finally, I shut up and let her ask all the sensible, practical questions that need to be asked. My answers almost make sense; they're half-formed at least. I'm planning to leave in just over a month, I'll be gone for a year, maybe more. I'll use the money I've saved up and borrow the rest. I have ideas for the first ten or so interviews and I'll go on from those once I get stateside.

As I hear her boil a kettle and ask if I have told the others, our old housemates, the reality of what I'm proposing starts to dawn on me. My reasons for the trip shift around in my brain. Am I doing this because I want to write a book, because I want to find the cause of stuttering, because I want to find role models for myself, or because I want to debunk the misconceptions around stuttering? What do I hope I'll find once I've spoken to all these people? Why do I want to immerse myself in stuttering when I have spent all of my life running away from it?

The adrenaline that has made me giddy in the wake of my decision is starting to wear off. I begin to doubt the whole plan. Can I really do this? Can I leave all my friends, my job, my whole life in London for some dream that I'm not sure will even work? How will I ever earn anything? Can I write at all? Should I take such a massive risk when I have a perfectly fine life in London?

My earlier bravado is shrinking drastically, chipped away with the emergence of each new doubt. "Buddy, this is really reckless and stupid, isn't it? Honestly, maybe I'm just losing my mind. Perhaps I'll wake up tomorrow and go back to work and put this whole thing behind me."

There's no pause. "No, no, not at all. I think it's brilliant, I think it is totally the right thing to do. But I'll miss you. We all will."

So will I. Desperately. And yet, despite my worries, I'm already planning what I will do when I land in America. I'm already hearing my parents' surprise, and I'm imagining the people I'll meet and the places I'll see. It doesn't feel like running away. It feels like the start of some new beginning that was lurking in my subconscious for a while. Maybe it is to do with stuttering, maybe not, but I have never been normal and I have never wanted a normal life.

As I tell Cat that I'll see her next week and hang up, I realize that there's one thing I haven't mentioned. One thing I expect I may not tell my parents, or anyone else, when I break the news over the coming weeks. I'm still holding out hope. I still think that if I can find the cause, then a cure is only one step away.

PART TWO

AMERICA

CHAPTER 8

TIGHTROPE OF LANGUAGE

Champaign-Urbana, January 2009

D R. LOUCKS'S SPEECH and hearing lab is not what I had imagined. Video cameras, microphones, and speech movement sensors have taken all the spaces that I expected to be filled with microscopes. Fiddling with a series of dials that would make a DJ proud, he motions towards a small earpiece on the counter.

It looks like a modern hearing aid, but I'm not so easily fooled. Growing up, I remember seeing the earpiece advertised in leaflets left lying around the house. The SpeechEasy device had been brought to the market by the Janus Development Group in 2001 and had been advertised as a miracle fix for stutterers. It worked on a principle I knew well: the idea that no one stutters when they speak in unison. I had read the brochures, I had learnt that the little electronic device used pitch shifting and something called delayed auditory feedback to echo my voice in an effort to re-create the choral effect in my brain. I knew that the little machines cost a staggering $4,000 to $5,000, depending on the model. I knew that my mum had brought the leaflets home because she wanted to help but, growing up, I had always seen them as a personal affront, as a reminder of all the ways that I was failing.

Despite my hesitation, I trust Dr. Torrey Loucks. He's a professor in the neurophysiology of stuttering at the Department of Speech and Hearing Science at the University of Illinois. He has spent the last hour patiently teaching me about the ways that stuttering is connected to the changeable, plastic chemistry of our brains. In the past few hours I have learnt that what we see as "stuttering" is really just a reaction; it is what our bodies are doing in response to something internal. The condition may be reflected in a motor act, but Dr. Loucks sees it as a motor sensory condition, trapped somewhere between the stage when we decide what to say and the moment when we burst our words forth.

"In terms of speech production, stuttering is interesting because it seems to fall at a junction that other speech disorders don't," explains Dr. Loucks. "It seems to arise after people have already formed what they intend to say. They have no issues in terms of forming properly grammatical statements: when they internalize their speech and when they speak to themselves, they don't stutter. Their brain is forming what they want to say, but the other part of their brain, the part that goes to execute what they want to say, is unable to carry it through."

Seeing the stutter as a motor glitch, as a physiological condition, makes it somehow less frightening, less of a personal failing.

"Slip on the earpiece. We're going to experiment with some different echo delays for a moment."

Gingerly I do as I'm told. I can't help but wonder if I'll be magically transported to some fluent landscape. He tells me that the optimal delay is just one-twentieth of a second and, as he decreases the delay to rest on the sweet spot, I start to read from a scientific textbook. At first I can hear my own voice calling after me. It sounds like a young child tugging at my sentences for attention, and then it speeds up and tramples over my words. I'm glad I'm reading rather than speaking spontaneously. It takes all my concentration not to be distracted by my phantom voice. I carry on speaking aimlessly until I become aware of myself. I have been almost entirely stutter-free. I'm impressed but not convinced. The distraction, the utter confusion is debilitating in its own way. I wonder if the effect will wear off soon enough, if the fluidity will fade as mysteriously as it arrived.

I look at Torrey and nod in tacit understanding. I assume it has worked how he was expecting. He is not an advocate of SpeechEasy but he studies the sensory-motor interactions of stuttering and the way SpeechEasy, though incompletely, affects those interactions.

"Great. I'll put it on now."

I can't understand why he is putting on the earpiece himself. It slightly annoys me. I know from speaking to him earlier that he is a fluent, "normal" speaker. He has no history of stuttering, and I'm not taken with the idea of his proving to me just *how* fluent he can be.

I watch him fiddle with some of the dials as he hums to himself. He changes the delay to a longer echo (known as long latency delayed auditory feedback) of a quarter of a second. Then he begins to speak and kidnaps my disinterest. The soft timbre of his Canadian accent is sullied, it becomes jagged and staccato as he blocks and ekes out his name. He takes off the earpiece and smiles warmly at my shock. "You see, Katherine, we all walk on a tightrope."

According to his research, some fluent speakers react by becoming more monotone, but approximately 20 percent (including himself) cannot produce even a short phrase without dysfluency. "The speech production system from brain to tongue can slide from fluency to dysfluency easily, but there is individual variation," explains Loucks. "Some have a solid, wide beam to walk across or they have superb balance. Others are a bit shakier and have a tendency to wobble more when circumstances are altered, such as delayed auditory feedback."

Poetry is not always visible in our everyday life. It is often hidden by the rough and tumble of surviving. The SpeechEasy device was not designed to reintroduce people to their humanity. It was created to mask stuttering and marketed as a virtual cure. Yet as I walk out of the lab and into the biting cold air of the Illinois winter, I don't feel like I need a crutch, I don't feel like a freak. Dr. Loucks has made me feel like a person sliding across the human spectrum. For the first time since I boarded the plane in London, I can see that all of us are standing together as we teeter on the edge of fluency and dysfluency.

• • •

ON OCTOBER 23, 2008, my plane landed at Boston's Logan Airport. My only plan was to get to my family's house in Cape Cod as soon as possible in order to map out the next year of my life. In the early 1980s, my dad had bought the wooden-shingled house as a holiday home, a place for my family to come every summer, a place to relax and spend time with his parents. As an American living in London, it was a way to keep a foothold in the country he had left behind, a way for his British family to learn about the world he had grown up in. As a child it had always been a refuge to me, a salt-encrusted place that hummed with the sound of crickets. He called it "our place of magic" and, in my final year of university, he had moved there for a job. Not wanting to leave me, her friends, or her home, my mum had stayed in England and visited him as often as possible. Gradually, her visits lengthened and she started to renovate the house, started to form a life for herself on the other side of the Atlantic. By the time I had landed in Boston, my parents were both largely living on the Cape, and I was moving home. When I returned as an adult, it was an easy place to think, a place to start working out where to begin.

Not yet bold enough to contact other stutterers, I started by reaching out to researchers and experts in the field. I wanted to know what caused stuttering, what made 1 percent of the world stutter while the other 99 percent only subconsciously thought of their speech. I wanted to meet pioneers and trailblazers face-to-face, to physically see their work and learn about their motivations. So I asked every stuttering association for their recommendations and got on the road. At first I stuck to the safety of the East Coast. I drove to Harvard, took the train to New York and the bus to Philadelphia. I flew down to Georgia and finally made the leap into the Midwest via Illinois. I carried my notes and my recorder from the National Institutes of Health, to the University of Illinois and the University of Pittsburgh.

Every person I met recommended another researcher and another therapist. I began to ask around for stutterers to interview. I wanted to find the truth behind stuttering. I expected that I might learn about the pain and the devastation it could bring about, but I also wanted role models, people who had decided to forge their path in the world, who had done exactly what they wanted despite their stutter. I wanted to meet stutterers who were smart and tough and courageous. I bought a map and began sticking pins in towns across America, places where I had heard there were interesting stutterers to interview. My pins ran the spine of the East Coast from Vermont down to Florida; they dotted across the Midwest and Southwest and finally snaked up the West Coast from Los Angeles to San Francisco. I gave myself ten months for more than a hundred interviews and planned for my research to culminate with the National Stuttering Association's annual conference in July.

At first the ten months seemed like a lifetime. Yet every stutterer I interviewed added another few recommendations to my list, and my notebooks started to strain at the seams, bursting with email addresses and phone numbers. To my surprise there were thousands of us, a disparate community of stutterers dotted across America.

I was shocked to hear people recommend actors, singers, news anchors, writers, and businessmen to speak to. Made bold and tenacious by my research, I hounded their publicists, their agents, and their secretaries to ask for an hour of their time. I reached out to celebrities whom I could never have imagined talking to, people who I had never realized stuttered. Some of my requests were rejected or ignored, but I was stunned at how many of them responded, how many of them invited me into their homes and their offices. I quickly saw how stuttering could be both a password and an equalizer.

Despite my excitement, homesickness did not take long to catch up with me. I took up everything from yoga to Toastmasters to keep my mind occupied during the dangerous breaks between frenzied days of research. Constant activity seemed to stave off the loneliness of travel, so I emailed my old housemates daily and called the other attendees of the Starfish project weekly. The more time I spent away from England, the harder it became. As the months passed, I longed for pub lunches, for weekends at Borough Market, for the drunken nights out in Henley that inevitably ended up with a dodgy kebab. I longed for my old friends.

Yet, as quiet as it was when I fell asleep every night, I was inwardly thrilled. I treasured the memories of my interviews, the moments when people allowed themselves to be blindly honest, the times that my small voice recorder seemed to disappear into the fabric of their homes. Finally my inquisitive nature, and my attraction to loaded, intimate conversations, was being used to the full.

The joy that I felt in the aftermath of my interviews became an amulet against the loneliness. I was fascinated by the ways people had handled their stutters, the difficulties they had faced, the way their speech had shaped their personalities, and the ways they had chosen to live their lives. I was thrilled to see that stutterers were standing in courtrooms, classrooms, hospitals, and on stages. It may not have been easy or painless, but they were not all hiding from a world that was scary to them. They upended my own misconceptions, and I realized that this book had the potential to topple so many of the fallacies that people held about stuttering and stutterers. We were not shy or nervous or stupid or weak. We may have been born with a different voice, but there was an important place for us in every part of the world.

I had no idea what would happen once I finished the interviews. I had no idea if I would go back to London to write and sell the book. I didn't have a plan beyond the belief that I was doing the right thing, that I was doing something necessary. I realized that I was trying to find out the truth of stuttering, to bring it out into the open, and stare at it for a while.

Our home in Cape Cod became my base, the place that I came back to whenever I needed to replenish my energy, hug my parents, and eat normally again. When I was traveling, I kept myself busy by transcribing my interviews on the long train rides and taking armloads of books with me on every flight. I collected books and articles and journals to learn about the history of stuttering and the study of speech. I quickly saw that the elusive search for a cause of stuttering had a rather long, and rather grim, history.

Having been first recorded in primitive hieroglyphs, stuttering was mentioned in biblical verses with Moses standing in front of the burning bush, pleading with God not to make him lead the Hebrews because he was "slow of speech and of a slow tongue." If the Bible was to believed, why had God chosen a stutterer to be his public speaking prophet? Did Moses' stutter make him more trustworthy or more courageous? What correlation did speaking truthfully, thoughtfully, and eloquently have to do with fluency? Beyond the Bible, the first mention of stuttering treatment came from a BC account of the Greek statesman and prominent orator Demosthenes reportedly overcoming his stutter, and strengthening his voice, by filling his mouth with pebbles and projecting his voice over the roar of the ocean.

Aristotle and his contemporary physicians saw the tongue as the center of the problem and prescribed everything from blistering afflicted tongues to wrapping them in towels. In the Middle Ages bloodletting and searing irons to the lips became the recognized treatments. By the nineteenth century even scarier theories had come to the forefront. The French physician Jean Marc Gaspard Itard had invented a fork made of gold or ivory to support the tongue during speech and was recommending gymnastic muscle exercises. In 1841 the Prussian surgeon Johann Friedrich Dieffenbach designed an operation (performed without general anesthesia) that involved cutting a deep wedge out of the sufferer's tongue. It seemed that everything had been attempted, including removing the adenoids, widening the dental arch, cutting a hole in the skull, and using appliances that prevented clenching, in order to keep the vital breathing passage open. I wondered if Dieffenbach had willing clients, if their desperation had made them fearless, or if they had been coerced.

I read that even the emergence of psychoanalysis in the early 1900s didn't leave stuttering untouched. Freud's devotees decided that stuttering must be caused by a mental imbalance and they traced it to everything from childhood trauma to sibling rivalry, suppressed anger, infantile sexual fixations, strict upbringing, and guilt. Even after those ideas were proven false, their theories managed to limp on regardless. Years later, even the brilliant film *The King's Speech* would indulge the tired misconception that a child's stutter could be caused by everything from an overbearing father to a sadistic nanny.

As my research led me into the modern day, it was clear that while experts knew that the disorder did not reside within the tongue or the larynx and was not caused by our upbringing, the true basis of stuttering was not yet fully understood. Despite its global prevalence and long historical lineage, stuttering seemed to remain an enigmatic condition with multiple causes. Much of the research I found classed stuttering as a multifactorial disorder and seemed to go no further. Then I discovered those who were working on the cutting edge of research, those whose investigations supported the idea that stuttering was a disorder of the brain.

In California, a physician called Dr. Gerald Maguire was both exploring the complex neurological pathways of stuttering and studying medical treatments. Having stuttered his whole life, in 1995 Maguire was part of the first team to use PET (positron-emission tomography) imaging scans to study the brains of people who stutter. His research proved that stuttering was associated with an abnormally low function of the left hemisphere of the brain, the area that was normally dominant in speech production. Maguire's research offered a clear explanation of why four times more men stutter than women. "Women can lateralize the right hemisphere better than men. They can be more right hemispheric dominant," he said. "So if the defect begins in a young girl, over time the little girl can actually develop a right hemisphere compensation for the left hemisphere."

Maguire believes that adults who stutter often have excessive dopamine in their brains, drawing strong similarities to Tourette's syndrome. Dopamine is the primary neurotransmitter that regulates motion, and surplus dopamine is strongly related to abnormally low functioning of the brain's striatum (a basal ganglia structure at the base of the brain). According to Maguire's research, the striatum performs as the brain's natural timer and initiator of speech, and he has researched medications that directly improve this central switchboard. Although there is currently no FDA drug approved for stuttering, Maguire has studied dopamine antagonists (approved for conditions such as Tourette's) that increase striatal function and relieve stuttering symptoms in many of his patients, including himself. He has personally experimented with many medications (everything from risperidone to olanzapine and ziprasidone), and is currently on asenapine. "Speech, with medication, has become automatic and natural to me. It used to be tiring and laboring to talk. Today, I don't monitor my speech anymore. I seldom think about the next word I'm going to say. If I stop the medication, in three days it is right back." According to his research 70 percent of his patients are helped by medication (30 percent see no change).

At the National Institutes of Health in Maryland, I met Dr. Dennis Drayna, a senior investigator at the National Institute on Deafness and Other Communication Disorders, and learnt that geneticists were examining whether stuttering could be a hereditary condition. In February 2010, a study by Drayna and his team of researchers pinpointed three gene mutations as the potential source of stuttering in volunteers in Pakistan, the United States, and England. The study stated that stuttering was possibly the result of a glitch in the day-to-day process by which cellular components in key regions of the brain were broken down and recycled.

"We are just beginning to uncover the underlying causes of stuttering, and most people don't think of it as a genetic disorder," explained Dr. Drayna. "But it turns out that a lot of people have put a great deal of work into this over many years and the evidence is really overwhelming that there is some genetic involvement. As a rough guess, about half of stuttering is due to genetic causes." Drayna and Maguire believe that, by pinpointing the cause of stuttering, we may see a dramatic expansion in our options for treatment. They passionately believe that we are on the precipice of a much deeper understanding of stuttering. Researchers have not yet discovered how the genes govern the problem but, in Maguire's emphatic words, "We have great genetic data, and we have the beginning of an understanding of a genetic marker. From there we can develop a target and a targeted medication to actually cure the underlying genetic defect at least for some individuals who stutter. The current forms of therapies are not cures, but I would not be accurate in saying that a cure would not be possible in my lifetime."

I felt relief in discovering that stuttering was wrapped up in the complex, plastic development of our brains. I was reassured to hear that, although stuttering may be subject to psychological influences, it was a complex, biological condition rather than a psychological hang-up. At the base of it, it was a relief to know that stuttering was not my fault, that it was not my parent's fault, or anyone else's. I had simply been born with a neuroanatomical weakness, nature had not chosen to give me effortless speech.

Yet, I could not completely share their enthusiasm. Although drugs had helped many, I was apprehensive to couple my own fluency to medications that were still in their infancy for stuttering. I was cautious to tie my hopes for success to a pill that had the potential for both side effects and disappointments. I felt dread in hearing that genetics accounted for more than 50 percent of stuttering cases. I had no history of stuttering in my own family. There may have been some hidden great uncle tucked away in some dusty family cupboard, but I had never heard of him. I had always believed that my stutter began and ended with me. I could accept passing on my miniature height, my tendency to overreact, even my inflexible stubbornness, but stuttering was an entirely different sort of gift to give. The thought that I could pass on my stutter to my unborn child was not entirely welcome information.

Still, I knew that I had never regretted my own birth. Even

in my darkest moments I had never wished not to be alive. As I traveled up to New York, I felt foolish to be worrying about something as distant as my theoretical unborn child. As single and carefree as I was, I knew that I wanted children eventually. It was easy to put my faith in the work of scientists such as Drayna and Maguire, and I suspected they would discover why 80 percent of kids spontaneously outgrew stuttering. I imagined that they might discover a cure within my lifetime. Still, I couldn't help but picture my theoretical child, a young, shy, blond-haired boy sitting alone on the school bus. I pictured him stuttering while asking the girl in front of him out on a date. I saw her shocked expression, heard her daunting laughter. Reflexively I shuddered.

"It was like a dagger through my heart when my son started stuttering," remembered big cat conservationist Alan Rabinowitz as we sat in his office overlooking Manhattan's Bryant Park. "Because the worst thing in the world was thinking he'd go through the unbelievable pain and agony I did. I had a horrible childhood because of it."

Would my child blame me for the defective genes I had passed on? Would he resent me? Worst of all, would I be ashamed by him?

There is a certain fear and guilt in seeing your child stutter for the first time. Many people who I interviewed remembered worrying that their child would have to experience all the same hurdles that they had faced. And yet, for those who did watch their children stutter into adolescence, there was a certain relief, an understanding that it would not be the nightmare they had feared. They told me of the bond they felt, the innate understanding that passed between parent and child. As human resources and organization development expert Jim Day explained, "I have a daughter who is now ten, and she has a very defined stutter. I prayed that she would grow out of it. But I now have a kinship with her and a certain bond because I get it. I'm glad I stutter because I feel I'm in a better position to help her. When I grew up I felt completely isolated and didn't have anyone to show me the ropes. I have a special solidarity with her that I don't have with my son."

Jim's words calmed some of my fears and ignited others. For the first time in my life, I worried about the possibility of having a fluent child. Would my child be ashamed of me? Would my stutter humiliate him? I remembered Michael Palin's candid account of growing up in a house made heavy by his father's stutter: "I'm sure I was embarrassed, but many times I just wished that he didn't have the stammer, it was as simple as that. I just wished that there was a magic wand that you could wave and the stammer would disappear." In strained, brutally frank words, Michael had remembered "feeling a sense of relief when I didn't have to listen to him." He remembered the tension that his father's short temper and frustration had put on their family: "I'm not saying that he was haunted by it, or that his life was ruined by it, but I think it must have been a great frustration. He was a good-looking man with a great sense of humor. He had a lot of things going for him, and yet this bloody stammer held him back. When I look back at his anger and his ill temper, it must have been his frustration."

I knew that frustration well, knew how my stutter could alienate people, knew how difficult it could be for others to witness my struggles. I knew that I had to talk about it, to put my stutter in its place, to work out how best to support myself if I was going to have any chance of putting others at ease. I wanted to be well placed to support any child I might have, especially if they stuttered, and yet I felt as if I was still working out how best to support myself. So I started to research what seemed to be working for others, what was on offer outside of traditional speech therapy and medication.

I was told of everything from vitamin supplements to hypnosis, relaxation classes, cranial osteopathy, and electric shock treatment. I read about courses that offered so-called cures at exorbitantly high prices. I heard everything from whispering in a delightfully phone-sex sort of voice to therapists who handed out gifts for fluent words in the spirit of positively reinforcing the stutter out of our voices.

None of the ideas appealed to me, but there were a handful of words that kept repeating over the monotonous bus rides and long train journeys. They had come from a gay North Carolinian journalist named Barry Yeoman, and they were hard to shake. "For forty years, gay people have been saying, 'We don't need to be pathologized, we don't need to be changed.' Now in stuttering groups, a lot of people are saying the same refrain."

What if there was nothing wrong with stuttering per se, what if we could somehow find some pride in our unique voices?

As I started to play with the idea of changing my attitude

rather than my speech, two ideas kept appearing again and again: voluntary stuttering and self-advertising. They came from the speech therapy world, but they were different from any other tool I had ever been taught. I learnt that the ideas had been pioneered in the 1950s by stutterer, researcher, and speech therapist Joseph Sheehan. Sheehan's therapy approach had been formed around four phases; one, the acceptance that we are stutterers and the creation of an open discussion around the subject; two, an increased awareness of what we do when we stutter; three, the seeking out of feared words and situations, and stuttering openly and easily; four, the development of a tolerance for dysfluency. Sheehan did not believe that stutterers should or could speak fluently, rather he believed that "only openness and honesty and a changing role of self-acceptance as a stutterer will lead to overcoming the tyranny of stuttering."

His theories and techniques had greatly influenced many of today's speech therapists, and I had first come across his focus on self-acceptance at Starfish. As part of the arsenal of tools we were given to keep our speech at bay, Anne had encouraged us to tell people that we were "proud recovering stutterers" and to stutter on purpose on words that we knew we could say fluently. I had watched people experiment with the ideas in the confines of the course and been impressed by stories of men and women standing in the supermarket and proclaiming their commitment to a speaking technique. I had sent my own email to my office telling them that I was working on my speech. Yet it was only in America that I saw what it meant to simply tell people that I stuttered. Not to say that I was working on changing my speech, but rather to stutter openly and to be proud of the voice I had. By early 2009, the idea of telling everyone I stuttered, and stuttering on purpose while doing it, had becoming both horrendous and magnetic.

As snow coated the streets of Midtown Manhattan, competitive pool player and marketing expert Steve Lipsky vividly remembered the first time that he went around the office of the Ithaca College Speech Language Program and told everyone that he stuttered, the first time he self-advertised: "It is such a cliché to say that it was the best day of my life and the worst day of my life, but the feeling of liberation was truly indescribable. I still get chills talking about it. It was a life-changing moment."

The high from those moments, the feeling of challenging yourself and being honest about who you are can be deeply addictive. Sitting in Philadelphia's 30th Street station, comedian Rob Bloom compared himself to someone who had battled alcoholism all his life. "Stuttering became my life. I told friends and family and everyone I could think of," he remembered. "I went through a phase where I would go up to people in the street. Every conversation would be prefaced by this disclaimer that I stuttered. It just completely consumed my life. I became 'Mr. Stutter'!"

Neither Steve's nor Rob's stories were unique. I met people who stood up on crowded subway cars to tell everyone that they stuttered, people who introduced themselves to strangers on the street and educated them on the complexities of the condition, people who wore T-shirts telling the world that they stuttered. I watched how they faced their biggest fears, how people laughed at them or turned and walked away, how they were not broken by their reactions.

As much as their stories inspired me, my British reserve balked against the idea of constantly shining the light in my direction to be praised or mocked. While self-advertising seemed too look-at-me-and-how-brave-I-am, pure voluntary stuttering appeared to be more quietly prideful.

At first glance voluntary stuttering seemed entirely counterintuitive. The idea was to stutter more, to stutter on purpose when talking to others in order to ultimately stutter less. The fluency was almost a byproduct rather than the goal. Much like self-advertising, voluntary stuttering built courage and combated shame. Above all, it let people take control of their speech. It gave them the power to manufacture a stutter while looking entirely relaxed. Done correctly, I could see how it could put speaker and listener at ease. Having spent his life rigorously hiding his stutter and fleeing from any word that might spell trouble, speech therapist Peter Reitzes remembered turning twenty-two unable to say anything at all. "I was so involved with avoiding stuttering that I had reached a point where anything I wanted to avoid would turn into a stutter." Under the advice of his therapist, he spent three and a half years stuttering on purpose and stuttering openly. When I met him he was working as a speech therapist in the Brooklyn public school system and looked like he was enjoying his speech. He seemed to barely notice any stutters that fell into his path. "Staying in the moment is a tough thing," he explained. "That's why I do voluntary stuttering, because when I do that, I give myself the permission to be there. I think being there is huge."

During my interviews in bars, restaurants, and hotels, I watched people stutter on purpose far more overtly than they would ever stutter naturally. I listened to people boldly play around with an entirely novel way of repeating and heard people use the tricky speaking techniques that they had learnt in therapy in the midst of a stutter that looked and sounded very real, but was their own conscious creation. They looked like they were enjoying it, and the whole concept sounded crazy enough to work.

I'M TERRIBLE at ordering coffee. I missed the memo when we were all told that getting a caffeine hit involved memorizing an entire new language. Standing inside a Boston Starbucks, I marvel at the woman ahead of me as she barks out her order. Apparently it is tall, skinny, dark, and topped with whipped cream. It sounds suspiciously like an advert from the back pages of the *Village Voice.* I would find the thought funny if I wasn't so scared.

As it is, I can feel every eye in the queue behind me boring into my back. My fingers are clenched, my chest is tight, and I'm silently willing myself to calm down. I shuffle forward and take my place in front of the cashier. She is wearing a headset and looks serious enough to be practicing surgery on my coffee order.

"What's your order?" she shouts at me as if I am standing on the other side of the café.

I have promised myself that I will throw in as many "hard"

stutters as I can muster. It is so simple. So ridiculously simple. I start the process and I realize how wrong I was.

"T t t t t t t ttt t t t ttt t ta ta ta ta."

I am stuttering in the same way I always do. I force myself to resist my natural inclination to apologize. My pretend stutter is almost identical to my "real" stutter and the two have morphed together and become monstrous.

Finally, I get out the word *tall*.

"A tall coffee?" The cashier is looking around nervously; I suspect that she is searching for an interpreter.

It would be so easy to just say yes. But I have promised myself that I'll do this.

"No, thanks. Just give me an ex ex extra moment here." I smile as confidently as I can. I take a deep breath and plan another fake stutter out in my head. I'll hiss the *s* out slowly and then block on the final word, I'll keep relaxed eye contact. If she looks away, I'll just stare at her shifting visor, "A t t t tall sssssssssssss soy l latte."

If I thought that my success would elicit a resounding high five from the cashier, I was sadly disappointed.

She has taken to shuffling behind the counter and replies with a slightly pitying, "Would this make it any easier?"

She's proffering a piece of paper and a pen. If there is any reaction more able to shatter my ecstasy, I'm hard-pressed to guess what it would be. I'm so caught up in the mounting emotion of the moment that I have to stop myself from snapping her pen in half.

And so I smile and I say, "No, thank you," as tightly as I can. She looks vaguely put out. "Are you sure?"

I can feel the line of customers shift awkwardly behind me.

Yes, I'm sure. I resume my request and viciously decide to pull the sentence out to its limits in punishment. The game is on.

"I'll say it again for you, so I'm sure you understand. IIIIIIIIII'll h h h h h h h h h h h h h have a tall sssssssssssss sssssssssssssssssssssssssssssssssssssssssssssssssssssssss soy latte."

For the first time in my life stuttering does feel like a game, like something I can play with. It feels malleable and controlled. Granted, the stutters do slip into the semi-real realm, but I am free of the fear of it.

For the first time in my life I can divorce the physical experience of stuttering from the anxiety. For the first time I can stutter without losing control, without caring about her reaction. I'm not unhinged by it.

I pick up my coffee victoriously. It is beautiful. Not because I have found a cure but because I have found something that feels right, something difficult and challenging that I can see making me feel good in the long run. It holds the potential for everyday victories rather than everyday defeats.

I am not going to be fluent. Who is?

CHAPTER 9

LOVE AS A MEDICINE

New York, January 2009

Describing Jeremy isn't easy. He seems to come out piece-meal, made up from a series of largely stolen glances.

"He has thick brown curls that he pushes back from his forehead, he's tall, he often looks thoughtful, but he has these dimples that soften his face. He's a year older than I am. He wears this woven bracelet that's really worn and tattered, and he has this striding way of walking, like he knows exactly where he's going."

I'm sounding like some besotted teenager. I can see it in Elektra's face as she smirks at me across the sitting room.

"Anyway, whatever, he's a sweet guy."

I glance back at the TV to shut myself up. Elektra breaks through the noise of the adverts. "So how did you meet this

179

wonder boy?" She is still smiling at me, like she knows a secret.

I am back in New York, staying at Elektra's flat for a few weeks. I've known her since I moved into her parents' spare room while interning in the city in 2005. Her mum was a friend of a friend back home in England, and they had offered to put me up for a couple of months while I earned next to no money. They had become my surrogate family in the city, and Elektra had become my streetwise guide.

Neither of us can sleep, and I'm not sure if I'm licking my wounds or pouring salt on them. I have just spent six short days with Jeremy in Chicago. I doubt I will ever see him again, so I am rehashing every moment of our very short relationship. Exercising every masochistic bone I have in my body.

"We met in Washington, DC, a couple months ago. I was down there with my cousin, researching this stuttering therapy called the McGuire Program and checking out one of their courses. Jeremy was there as an alumnus, helping the first timers and encouraging them to use the techniques." I pause for a moment. I want to keep my cool, but I'm not quite ready to stop remembering. I can still see the easy smile he shot in my direction when I caught his eye. I can still hear the rolling sound of his voice as he gently encouraged me to join the group exercises. I force my voice not to betray any of my foolish excitement. "I only met him for a couple of hours and we barely exchanged a few sentences, but there was something about him. So I asked for his number."

Her eyebrows shoot up.

"That's the joy of writing a book. When I ask a guy for his phone number it is usually to plan an interview, so I look like a diligent reporter rather than a crazed stalker. Who knew writing a book would be such a great way to meet men!" I'm trying to lighten the anvil in my stomach. It works for a second.

She's not so easily deterred. "So you called him?"

"Not exactly." Not at all, if I'm honest. I had found the courage to ask for his phone number, but my confidence had faltered from that moment on. I had looked at his number in my phone a couple of times and thought about calling, but a phone call felt dangerous. It was more loaded with past and present worries, for both of us. When I had met him in Washington, Jeremy's voice was trained, bent to his will by the same structured speaking technique that I had learnt at Starfish. We both stuttered, but he was battling for fluency, keen for a new voice. I was well aware that my decision to speak spontaneously went against his resolve. I worried that my voice on the phone might scare him away. Worried that he was trying to get as far away as he could from a voice like mine.

"He called me two months after we met. Out of the blue he called to ask if I was still interested in interviewing him. He wanted to let me know that there was a flight sale to Chicago in early January."

I can't help but smile foolishly. "So, crazy as I may be, I went. I jetted off to see a man who was, for all intents and purposes, a total stranger. But I was all business, I had other interviews lined up, I was focused."

She raises her eyebrows again.

"Well, I was for the first few days. Then, my focus shifted." I could remember how serious I was when I arrived at Chicago's O'Hare Airport, how determined I was to prepare for my interviews, how quickly my resolve to type up my transcriptions every evening had waned. Work had struggled to compete with offers to go ice-skating or listen to the blues. I remembered the first time we kissed, the first time we stayed up all night talking. I could feel the familiar giddiness muddy my thoughts. Luckily, I know that I'm reserved enough to keep them to myself. "I couldn't help it. Jeremy just knows Chicago so well, and he cheered up a friend by taking her tobogganing, and he introduced me to his dad . . ."

Despite my best attempts to keep my cool, I can hear myself start to ramble. I stop talking and let myself give in to an irrepressible grin. Elektra sips her tea and looks at me suspiciously for a few seconds.

"So what's the problem?"

"First of all, I left Chicago before anything had really begun."

"You had to, you're researching a book. You can't just give up because you meet some guy."

"I know, I know. But there's more." I pause. I know that I probably sound completely crazy so I try to start off as rationally as I can. "There are so many people I want to interview in the Southwest and on the West Coast. So I have been planning out this ss s s s sss s s ix-week road trip ac ac ac ac across the country from T t t t t ttt t t texas to California, and I decided that I didn't want to do the jour jour jour jour journey alone, that I wanted to do it with him." As always my voice is exposing my disappointment, my breathless nerves, my embarrassment. "So last night I sent him an email asking if he wanted to do the trip to to to to to to together. Now it has been ages and I haven't heard anything. I have probably scared him off for good."

Elektra looks at me in silence for a moment. I don't have the energy to convince her, or myself. "You're mad." She says it smiling, but I sense she is right. I sense that I have lost my sanity. I hear her reassure me that it is probably fine, that it has only been twenty-four hours, that I should stop worrying. I wish I believed her. I keep glancing at my phone and pretending to watch the TV.

That evening ten o'clock rolls into eleven, and then my phone starts to glow blue. It vibrates off the small coffee table. I scramble to pick it up, hyperventilate gracelessly for a few brief seconds, slide into the bedroom next door, and then answer. "H H H H H H H H H H ello."

"H H hi there." I can hear him smiling on the other side of the line, and I picture him leaning against his apartment's wooden porch. I sit down on the bed. I can feel myself breathing a little less frantically. After all, I realize that it is his voice that I have missed most of all, the only part of him that I hadn't mentioned to Elektra.

"So this road trip sounds like a wonderful adventure. Tell me all about it."

A STUTTERING couple is a rarity, a novelty to be met with questions, sage nods, and puzzled brows. In my years of meeting other stutterers, I have only come across one other couple. Today I'm not entirely surprised. The path is not as easy as I once thought. I'm well aware of both the beauty and the difficulty of falling in love with each other.

From the outside it seemed easy, the easiest thing in the world, to feel close to someone who shared something so elemental. We planned our road trip quickly, both excited to be together again. I traveled down to Texas a week early for ten interviews in Dallas and Houston. As I interviewed everyone from a former San Diego Chargers quarterback to a neurologist and a personal trainer, Jeremy bought a Subaru Outback in Dallas and drove to meet me in Houston. Finally, less than a month after we had said good-bye in Chicago, we set off on the road together.

At the outset of our adventure we spent four days camping in Texas's Big Bend National Park. In the silence of the endless desert, free from the reactions of the rest of the world, we were able to dream a little. We read books to each other and told stories over the long hikes. I heard about his dad's used book store, about the friends he treasured from his years at Whitman College, about his adventures around the world. Gradually his words slipped into the loaded territory of our speech.

He told me how he had marginalized himself in the past, how he hadn't spoken up or sought opportunities because he had told himself that he couldn't do certain things. He remembered how things had begun to change in his late teens, how he had started to volunteer, to travel, and to do the things that scared him the most. He had joined Toastmasters and confronted his stutter at the McGuire Program. As he remembered the mean songs that schoolkids had made up to mock his stutter, he explained how being bullied had motivated him to succeed, how it had fostered a belief that if he was anything less than wildly successful it would prove them right. It had driven him to be self-sufficient from a young age, to buy and renovate houses across the country, and to earn enough money to start his own business. He was excited about the life he had, and yet he was striving to do better, to bring more to the table. He wanted to learn more, to be more, to spend more time with the people he loved. As I listened to his stories and watched him stutter, I saw how courageous it made him, how attractive I found it. He was never made ugly by it, never even close.

Over the course of my interviews I had seen beautiful marriages between stutterers and their fluent partners. I had watched wives stare at their husbands in open admiration as I interviewed them, I had listened to husbands tell me stories of their wives' various talents. I had seen women openly glare at any waitress who mocked their partners' speech. I had seen plenty of proof that stuttering was not unattractive. Yet I had also heard horror stories.

A man I interviewed in Sea Island, Georgia, had been married for more than thirty years. He was still married to his wife, but she didn't let him call her at work for fear that someone would find out that he stuttered. She told him that he needed to get fixed, that he could not accept himself as a stutterer. I wondered why she married him, why he married her. It shocked me, and I felt a twinge of guilt.

Until I met Jeremy, I had never even thought of going out with someone who stuttered. My reasoning was entirely selfish. I had no urge to look in the mirror every day. I took safety in the knowledge that no one entirely understood the complicated, ugly depths of my feelings towards my speech. With Jeremy there was no room for hiding anymore, no room for secrets. Instead, there was a plain, unspoken understanding that took little more than an eye roll or a smile to explain. There was a connection that was both comforting and disarming. I began to see how our relationship could be strained by the empathy that drew us together.

I had planned interviews scattered across the Southwest and, on our road trip across the country, we had "couch surfed" in various small towns and villages to save money. Having never heard of couch surfing before meeting Jeremy, he introduced me to an entirely new form of traveling. With our very limited budget, couchsurfing.org offered a way for us to stay with locals, for free, wherever Jeremy didn't have friends. I was skeptical at first, wary of the motives of these oddly hospitable strangers, but my bank balance and Jeremy's company persuaded me to become a member. We composed our online profile, wrote about the journey we were on, looked for hosts with positive references in each area, and requested to stay on their couch or spare bedroom (when we were lucky).

It meant that we arrived at a stranger's house in each new town, stayed for a couple of nights, and moved on. We were constantly introducing ourselves, constantly speaking to people we had never met. We were constantly seeing what others saw in us, the strangeness of two stutterers on an odyssey together.

Stuttering lends an intensity to conversations that makes you more engaged and makes superficial banter tricky. When you talk to someone who stutters, you are forced to concentrate more and to listen more actively. When someone stutters, they throw their energy into speaking so it makes sense that their audience would do the same. I knew that I felt drained at the end of a particularly dysfluent day, I knew that when I listened to a person blocking and repeating, I felt as if I were physically fighting for them. I imagined that our hosts might have felt the same, that they might have been exhausted at the end of an evening with us.

I had spent much of my life controlling myself, controlling when I spoke, who I spoke to, and how I responded to the reactions I saw. As NYU oncology nurse Roisin McManus explained, "I can't control anything about what someone else does and how they feel." Roisin was part of the only other stuttering couple I had ever met. She remembered how she had to give up the control that she had fought to maintain for so long, "It was a good thing, to give it up, a positive thing to do. But I really thought about it." Dating Jeremy forced me to let go entirely; it forced me to let the chips fall and not to fret about the outcome.

I had my own roadblock style of stuttering. On particularly challenging days I could feel an invisible wall emerge in the middle of every word. I would start over and run up at the word enough times to push it out. I would repeat certain sounds that seemed to stick resolutely in my chest. I would feel dizzy and tight in expectation of the difficulty to come.

Jeremy had his own unique way of speaking that was entirely his own, entirely different from mine. When he stuttered, it sounded thoughtful, as if he were searching for the word he wanted through a series of barely noticeable "ums" and "ahs." He looked like he was in the middle of some cerebral process. Very rarely he would block, and it would seem to open his eyes, to freeze him momentarily, until the word popped out intact.

Ultimately, being with him felt like stuttering for two, it meant tacking his style onto my own. I could feel the familiar deep breath and reverberation of his speaking technique. I could feel him strain to make himself pause in the middle of a sentence. As he went into a block, I would feel the familiar breathlessness travel up my throat. I could taste his stutters as he laid them out across the air. I could watch him and see how he assessed a room, how he waited for the right moment to speak, how he said whatever he wanted. I took on his speech and his nerves and his fearlessness as if they were my own. I saw him do the same. We worried about each other, worried how the other was feeling, worried about others' reactions.

In a coffee shop in Taos, New Mexico, I explained the journey that I was on and asked the cashier if she knew anyone in the area who stuttered. I watched her face transform into a grin, heard her reply that she didn't know any stutterers, that she didn't have anyone to make fun of. I felt Jeremy stand behind me, felt him lean forward, heard the deep rumble of his voice as he told her that she must not be a very funny person, that she must have a terrible sense of humor if she needed to make fun of stutterers. I heard his cold, charming smile and felt the air move as he swept away to ask some of the café customers if they knew of anyone I could interview. In the midst of her groveling apologies I felt proud, bolstered, and in awe of this straight-talking American I had by my side.

Although I had to deal with my own anxiety, I never wanted to change Jeremy. I was never embarrassed by him, never wished that he was fluent. On the road trip I started to realize that Jeremy filled the hole that had been missing in my life. Over the endless miles of open country we started to piece together some unknown future.

I could no longer picture my life without him, yet I had questions, black holes that needed to be filled in my rose-tinted vision of our life together. Luckily, Jeremy was the first man that I met who complemented my emotional outbursts and interrogations. He was the first person who shared my vulnerabilities and my frustrations, the first person who justi-fied and lessened them. He was spontaneous and loving and practical and interesting. Endlessly interesting. He was never reserved and always honest. I could ask him anything.

As we drove through the soaring towers of Monument Val-ley, I asked him if my stutter made him uncomfortable. "It did at first. I had been on a speech program where everything was very regimented, and I was caught off guard at somebody so beautiful, with so much going for her, who chose to stut-ter openly." The burnt scenery carried on past the window silently, "Now you are my whole view of the world. It is just who you are."

Making our way across the desolate Arizona desert late one night, I explained how it felt like he was sometimes run-ning away from his stutter and crashing into me. He nodded for a moment. "It's true." He paused. "It makes me feel very vulnerable." I could have left it there, but I could feel the next question pressing at my lips, forcing itself out. "What if we have kids who stutter? What will you think of them? How will you react?"

The thought had been in my head for a while, I assumed that our chances were pretty high, but I couldn't believe that I had asked it, couldn't believe I had assumed so much. Blanketed by the darkness, I pinched my arm to stop any more pronoun-loaded words tumbling out. The hum of the engine and the wheels skimming the tarmac filled the resulting quiet. I knew that his answer was coming, knew that I needed to be patient. He was the first person to teach me to appreciate silence, one of the few people I knew who was not afraid of taking the time to craft his words carefully. The minutes ticked by and, while he thought, I let myself imagine my own answer.

I wouldn't rush them; I would listen; I would laugh at their jokes; I would have high expectations of all they could achieve; I would urge them to speak up; I would teach them the importance of eye contact; I would remind them that, even on their "worst" stuttering days, life still goes on; I would never shame them; I would teach them to gravitate towards generous people who would do the same; I would frame therapy carefully, keep it away from the loaded words of "cure" and "fluency." I was deep in thought when his answer came, his eyes still focused intently on the rear lights of the cars ahead, "I, or we, hopefully, will love them completely for who they are, for each way that they are unique." He paused again, and I wondered if he was finished. Then he glanced at me and grinned while he squeezed my hand, "Plus, who could ask for better parents?"

His answer was all that I hoped it would be. And he was right, I was sure that he would make an incredible father. His answer enveloped me and rocked me to sleep as we drove into San Diego. Days later, my subdued anxiety returned with a strength I no longer thought it had. Tired and irritable after a day spent driving in Los Angeles, I vented the frustration that had been festering in the midday heat. I asked why he sometimes wouldn't look me in the eye when I stuttered, why he seemed impatient or ashamed. He looked crestfallen for a moment, and I instantly regretted asking. I was sure that I had done the same, sure that he had never meant to hurt me. Finally, we pulled off the highway and stopped. "Katherine, I love you. But you don't need me, or anyone else, to validate you."

That was it. That was the moment I stopped. In the resulting calm I stopped questioning him, stopped questioning his feelings. He loved me, we were both perfectly imperfect, and he was right, of course. None of us needed to be given the okay by others, none of our happiness was dependent on someone else. I wanted to stop myself from caring about what others thought, but my stutter had made me hyperaware of the world around me. I was starting to escape the judgment of the rest of the world, but it was taking time.

I'M STARING at the pages of the Haggadah. I hope that I look impressively interested in the words. Truth be told, I'm counting the lines until Gene stops talking and the readings start to wind their way around the table. I haven't counted pages since I was sixteen. I remember my old tricks. How I would slip off to the bathroom at an opportune moment or tell my

teachers that I had a sore throat, that reading would be difficult for me. I remember how they had all played along kindly
with the charade. For a brief second I contemplate both options and Jeremy's hand seems to get hotter on my knee.

I look up at Gene, an old friend of Jeremy's parents, and it
is clear that the seder means a great deal to him. It is the first
time I've ever taken part in any Jewish traditions, and I taunt
myself with thoughts of how he will feel if I ruin his well-
planned ritual. To calm myself I take my eyes away from the
text. I stare out the window at the white-crested waves of Lake
Michigan. I look back at the food overflowing on the table and
the yarmulkes leaning towards me from the top of the men's
heads opposite me. I catch the eye of Jeremy's mum, and she
smiles at me encouragingly. I try to arrange my face into a
relaxed grin, but I feel it turn to a grimace as I realize the next
person is talking. All too soon it will be Jeremy's turn, and
then mine.

I had met Jeremy's parents months ago in San Francisco,
months before I had moved in with Jeremy in Chicago. I had
asked him what they would think of me, what they would
think of the mysterious girl who had kidnapped their son for
almost two months. I need not have worried. They were re-
markably thoughtful and caring. The sort of people who were
quick to cry and quicker to laugh. The sort of people I wanted
to like me.

I know that they will never judge my stutter, that they
have navigated Jeremy's speech all his life. But I wonder what
they think. I wonder if they find it strange. I wonder if they
ever wish for an easier, less loaded conversation. I watch as

his mum reads her piece, I see how she deftly enunciates the heavy Hebrew. I listen to the woman adjacent to her begin.

Jeremy's turn is next, and then mine. I am nervous for him, hoping that he will get through it unscathed. I am already berating myself for my future stuttering, already going through the palpitations of each unspoken block. I wonder what will happen if I block painfully for long minutes. Wonder if everyone will look down awkwardly or if someone will decide to rescue me and embarrass me further. The voice in my head tells me to calm down, that I'll be fine. Nothing terrible will happen if I stutter, or if Jeremy stutters. Nothing miraculous will happen if we are fluent. Jeremy squeezes my knee. I love him for it but don't want to know that he is aware of my nerves. I don't want to think that this might be difficult for him. I need him to comfort me, want to comfort him, and resent that need.

Then the woman stops talking and there's silence. Jeremy's turn has arrived. My own fears go mute and I just hope that he will be okay. I feel him squeeze my knee again, and I lay my hand over his.

"Would it be okay if we did our readings together?"

I can't tell if he's asking me or the table. Surprise renders me speechless. I nod my head and he smiles. "Thanks." As if it's the easiest thing in the world, as if I'm doing him a big favor.

So we read, in unison. Together each syllable comes out intact and strong. It is a beautiful defeat. I have not faced my fear, neither of us has felt the nervous adrenaline flood our voices. We have chosen not to take the gamble, this time. We have chosen to take it easy. Jeremy knows that neither of us will ever falter if we read together. I suspect that his offer may be laced with embarrassment, but it is born of compassion and kindness. He knows that it is the one way he can protect us both.

For the rest of the meal we talk easily to everyone around us. I stutter openly, throw in some voluntary stutters, I watch Jeremy do the same. Nothing has changed, but there's a complicity to it. A winking sort of understanding that we are working something out. It may be difficult at times, it won't always be easy, but we're in it together.

I remember how the writer Ted Hoagland told me that love conquered his stutter, that when he was in love with a woman he could speak with her completely fluently. Love does nothing to my speech, but I can see that loving Jeremy makes me feel comfortable with being uncomfortable, comfortable with looking in the mirror. Or at least it did. Today I no longer see Jeremy's stutter, or at least I no longer see it apart from him. I still smile at him if I hear a block or laugh if both of us are having trouble with a particular word. But his voice is his, it does not fit any labels, it is just who he is. It is one of the many pieces that I love about him.

Whatever stuttering has taken away I realize that it has introduced me to Jeremy. If I can love him so completely then I suspect I can do the same for myself.

CHAPTER 10

ROLE MODELS

Scottsdale, July 2009

Y OU HERE FOR the stuttering conference?"

She makes it sound like I am there to be taught *how* to stutter, how to improve the delivery of my repetitions and really lengthen my blocks. I wonder what the three people in line behind me think. I assume that the two men must be in Scottsdale for some business meeting. Unkindly I dismiss the woman. With her cascading brown hair, I assume that she is the pampered and preened type who will lie by the hotel's pool while her husband spends his days trapped in the air-conditioned conference rooms.

I lean away from them, towards the hotel concierge. "I am. I'm here for the National Stuttering Association conference." I pause for a moment. I'm tempted to explain to her what the

NSA is all about, how it is born out of the self-help movement, how it is a chance for stutterers to get together and learn from each other. But, in all honesty, I'm intrigued how she knows that I'm here for the conference, wondering whether I somehow look like a stutterer to her. "How did you know?"

She continues typing furiously on her hidden computer. "Some guy called Jeremy Cohen has upgraded you both to one of our suites."

Of course. I can imagine Jeremy doing it. I can see him slipping the lady a twenty as he shakes her hand and asks her if she has a really wonderful room for us. I smile at her as she hands me the key. It is the first time that she has looked at me. I wonder what she'll do with the cash later.

As I move away from the counter the heat slips in from the front door and renders the air-conditioning useless. It is late afternoon and the Arizona heat is still strong, still oppressive. I turn to go towards the elevator bank and hear the men behind me in line start stuttering. I watch the brunette stomp her foot and throw back her head as she tells the receptionist her name. I hear the two older women sitting in some nearby seats regale each other with their flight mishaps. I see two young women run up to each other and see a family holding hands as they stand awkwardly in the periphery of the lobby.

Everyone is stuttering.

I can't hear a fluent word. I feel like I have stumbled upon some alternate universe where stuttering is the norm. I was expecting it and yet it stops me for a moment.

"Katherine." I can hear a familiar voice, a couple of voices. "Katherine, we're down here."

Being short-sighted is unhelpful at the best of times. I wave in the general direction of the voices. I can see some long brown hair, a short blond bob, a taller body, and some gray hair. As I walk towards them they come into focus. There's Caryn, a speech therapist in her midtwenties with an infectious laugh. There's Russ, a white-haired Texan and expert Toastmaster who speaks nonstop; Samantha, a media specialist living in New Jersey; and Joel, who regularly cohosts the popular podcast *Stuttertalk* from his home in Minneapolis. Then there's Jeremy, waving at me as he leans against the bar.

As I walk towards them I can see them giggling at a joke I can't hear. I smile in anticipation. The place is heaving with bodies. As I squeeze through the bar, I wave at more familiar faces, hug more of the people that I interviewed. I catch pieces of their conversations. I hear them congratulate each other at getting the extra time off work. I piece together half-formed sentences as they sip their drinks and tell each other that the annual conference is the highlight of their year.

It is the first time that I've heard so many stutters in one place, and I'm transfixed by the cacophony. There are rapid-fire machine gun–style syllables, broken sentences, rap-style repetitions, blocks that disappear into the end of breathless words. There are stutters that I barely notice and those that demand my attention. There are people who seem to love speaking and those who look like they are battling for their piece in the conversation.

When I finally make it to the group, I throw my arms around everyone as I listen to Jeremy tell the end of an old joke. The group starts laughing and Eric, a banker turned speech therapist in his early thirties, starts on his own story as I rest on the bar to get the barman's attention. "I'd love a g g g g g g g g gin and tonic." The bartender smiles, nods, and begins to pour as I fumble for my purse and ask around if anyone's drink needs refilling.

"You know, I had a stutter growing up, too," the bartender seems anxious to tell me. I smile. I feel like I'm congratulating him. I wonder if he's keen to be incorporated into the group. I look over at the motley crew of young, successful, funny stutterers. It is the sort of group I imagine someone might want to belong to, the sort of group that I can feel myself being pulled into. Eric overhears him and shouts out, 'Hey, that's awesome, man, you're one of us." He beams in his direction. Apparently not only is it just okay to stutter—a badge of honor.

It takes me some time to get used to the idea. The NSA annual conference is the largest gathering of stutterers in the country. Along with similar organizations like Friends (aimed at children) and the British Stammering Association in England, its mission is not to provide speech therapy, but rather to give support and education to people who stutter. The self-help jargon of the conference's pride-laced conversations grate against my natural skepticism. I come from a background of self-effacement, and all the clapping praise makes me feel awkward. Yet in the surreal confines of the hotel's walls, I feel myself gradually change. There's a deep sense of comfort that is rarely sustained in the grittiness of the real world. I stop thinking about my speech, I stop listening out for my own stumbles. I watch as a group of kids give a speech at a podium for the first time in their lives and see their parents tear up in reply. I use more voluntary stuttering because I feel comfortable playing with my speech, because I want to stutter.

And yet, I can see that the joy of the conference is tinged with something a little darker. I hear about broken families and broken dreams, I realize that, for many, the NSA is the only place they feel entirely accepted. Jacksonville accountant Bob Wellington puts it best: "The one thing that I have carried throughout my life is the sense of not fitting in." In his words, "The NSA is a place that I can feel accepted, a place that I know is safe, and a place that I may be able to call home, for the first time in my life."

Speech therapist and conference veteran Caryn Herring jokes that the majority of her friends are stutterers. "While I am very comfortable and very open with my stuttering at this point in my life, being around other people who stutter is the only time when hiding or avoiding stuttering is never even considered." As she puts it, "Surrounding myself with people who stutter helps me remember that I'm not alone."

IT SEEMS that stutterers are far from the freaks and outcasts that I once pegged them to be. They are different, certainly different, but, in the words of Alan Rabinowitz, "Stutterers are very special people indeed." As he explains, "I find stutterers to be more sensitive, much more driven. I mean, you could go either way, you could become a serial murderer being driven. But generally the stutterers I have known are very driven people who go overboard at succeeding." They see the world from a different perspective and they tend to have a thrust behind them that validates them.

Stutterers are not saints. I'm not arguing that we are somehow better than everyone else. My world is not solely composed of stutterers, and most of my closest friends and family are fluent speakers. In my year of interviews, I met some stutterers who shocked me, people who were dogmatic and rude and boring and mean. I also met more people I liked, more people whom I felt at ease around, more people who could become role models for the way that I wanted to live my life.

Growing up, I had no stuttering role models. Until my twenties, the film industry had not cast a stutterer in the role of the hero. If Hollywood was anything to go by, I assumed that heroes had to be strong, fearless, and assertive. I strained my mind to imagine how a stuttering character would fit into that mold.

But, as I spoke to my final few interviewees in the aftermath of the NSA convention, I could clearly see that stutterers could be strong and confident. They could be the quintessential heroes that I had in my mind's eye. It seemed that they became heroic because they refused to accept normalcy, because they wanted more, because they had something to prove to the world. In the words of film director Jeff Blitz, "I'm not going to stay in the box that the indifferent universe has put me into."

There were heroes like GE legend Jack Welch, actress Emily Blunt, and the effortlessly cool singer Bill Withers. As inspiring as they were, they came later in my journey. The first idol that I met was writer and big cat conservationist

Alan Rabinowitz. Alan told me that he believed that animals helped him as a child because he could talk to them, because they were his only friends. "I swore, if I could ever control my stutter, I would use it for them and that's how I ended up following my life." Today he is a fearless Indiana Jones figure, the darling of everyone from *The Colbert Report* to *National Geographic.* "It is because of stuttering that I don't just study jaguars, but that I have to set up the world's first jaguar preserve, I have to set up the world's largest tiger reserve. I have to save these animals, but I also have to save myself. Those two will never be apart."

Alan remembers a childhood of being called a retard and admits that, even today, he can never escape the little stuttering boy inside of him, that none of us can. "As much as I spent my whole life trying not to care what people think, I still care. That's why I'm always looking for accolades. I truly love what I do, but I also want people to say, 'You're so great.' It doesn't have anything to do with money or anything; it has to do with that little stuttering boy who nobody thought could amount to anything."

Alan's story is unique, but it expressed a sentiment I heard over and over on my travels. After eighteen years climbing the corporate ladder at a pharmaceutical company, Sander Flaum remembered the moment that he was finally up for the prestigious general manager position. Human Resources had heavily hinted that he was the favorite and he was crushed to hear that the board had not chosen him. In his angry disappointment he left. He had led every top division and was baffled by their decision. Months later he found out the reason. The assistant general manager asked him to lunch to explain. He told him that one of the board members had convinced everyone that stuttering was symptomatic of mental illness, that he could not be trusted, that it would be too much of a risk to give him a job because he was a stutterer. "It was incredibly difficult for me to hear that," remembers Sander. "A few months afterwards, I got a call to come back to the company on a huge salary increase. I just turned it down. I said, I'm not going to do it and my goal is to become more successful than anybody there. And then that was what I did."

I heard about many people who were successful in order to prove something to themselves and to others. The most powerful heroes I met were the ones who were not cured but not cowed either. The people whom I most admired were the ones who saw their stutter as an asset, those who could see the talents and the perspective that their speech gave them.

Roisin McManus, an oncology nurse at NYU's medical center, works with patients who are in very vulnerable situations; some are chronic and others are stuck in the hospital for months on end. "Stuttering may not be a terminal illness, but it gives me more understanding of the depths that people can go to when something difficult is placed on them," she explains. "I have an idea of where a challenging situation can take people. Stuttering took me to hiding in a bathroom in high school, so if someone is being really needy or really mean, I don't always know what they're dealing with, but I know that we can't always be together. I know that we can't always be intact."

As a kid I believed that my life would be perfect if I didn't stutter. I never considered that my stutter might make me better, I never thought that I could excel in a field not simply in spite of my stutter but because of it. Barry Yeoman believes that stuttering makes him a better journalist because he is less intimidating, he loves to listen, and he has a natural empathy for underdogs. Singer and guitarist Chris Trapper is a successful musician, a man who comes into his own onstage. He worries that, if his stutter ever disappeared, it may take something more precious along with it. "It would change the way that I express myself. I worry about losing my songwriting, my whole income, my whole life, my whole identity really."

Stuttering ensures a deep appreciation of the beauty of words and language. As Jeff Blitz, the writer-director of the movie *Rocket Science* (an award-winning film about a young stuttering boy who joins a high-school debate team), puts it, "You discover that words have a certain kind of power and you become much more intimate with how they sound." When I speak, my sentences are fought for and my words burst forward. When I speak my rhythm is at the whim of my stutter, at times it surges forward and at times it crashes. My stutter ensures that when I put the effort into speaking, I make sure that I'm saying something worthwhile. The difficulty of speaking forces stutterers away from glib small talk. "I work out, I've got really developed jaw muscles," laughs Jamie Rocchio. "It hurts me to stutter. My jaws ache and I'm exhausted at the end of the day. It takes a lot out of me to talk, so I'm not going to talk idly."

Writing is less exhausting than speaking. For me it is both an obsession and an addiction. On the page I try to give myself the graceful voice that often eluded me in real life. Writing fulfills my fantasy of verbal control. "I feel like so much of what drives me as a writer has to do with a revenge on stuttering," explains writer David Shields. "It is not only that it fed my desire to be a writer, but it fed my desire to be a writer with a relatively characteristic and idiosyncratic voice."

"What does a stutterer do? What can you possibly do in a society like this?" asks Harvard professor Marc Shell. "You can become a writer." There may be a whole slew of careers at a stutterer's disposal, but it can be no coincidence that stutterers have a long literary history. I had always dreamed of becoming a writer. And yet, as I delved into the history of stuttering, I realized that we had a more impressive lineage than I had ever imagined. Somerset Maugham wrote because he didn't want to speak, and Lewis Carroll was held back from the priesthood because of his stutter. I wondered whether the literary style of Henry James, John Updike, David Mitchell, Margaret Drabble, and Philip Larkin was affected by their stuttered speech, whether their talents were cultivated in the hours they spent observing and thinking rather than talking. I interviewed men who had chosen to make their condition part of their body of work. Marc Shell, David Shields, Benson Bobrick, Ted Hoagland, and Alan Rabinowitz discussed the subject in memoirs, pseudofictional characters, and treatises.

I suspected that, for all of us, writing was a necessary outlet for our screaming internal dialogues. I knew that my stutter had, in large part, pushed me towards becoming a writer. I also saw how it could sustain me, how it could carry me through the less pleasant moments. Over the years I had hardened myself against any rejections I might see in the eyes of my audience. I was difficult to humiliate. As Ted Hoagland explains, "As a stutterer you have to grow a carapace because your feelings are going to be hurt, there are going to be people who pick on you and are rude to you, you have to be able to survive blows." I was hardened and striving to prove myself worthy. As I sat down to write this book, I felt I had a story to tell but was well aware that it might be a path paved with a fair amount of risk and a lot of rejection.

By the time the four-day NSA convention ended, I had spent ten months interviewing more than a hundred stutterers, speech therapists, and researchers. It was time to return home. Not to Jeremy's house in Chicago or my home in England, but to my family's place on Cape Cod. I was looking forward to moving in with Jeremy in October, but first I wanted to return to the house that I had known all of my life, the one place old enough to hold all my memories. After almost a year of traveling, I transcribed all of their voices sitting amongst the familiar furniture. As I typed hundreds of hours of words, I sat in the imprint of my grandma's armchair and slid my feet in and out of the worn topsiders that my dad had bought me to celebrate my first sailing lesson.

As I strained my ears to catch the unique cadence of each stuttered word, I heard the clock that my grandpa had built chime away the hours. As the end-of-summer heat slipped in from the deck, I felt my skirt flutter and remembered the excitement I had felt buying it, of slipping the fresh silk around my legs after a month spent in dirt-encrusted clothes backpacking around Thailand when I was twenty-two. There were pictures scattered around the house, too: all my university housemates grinning wildly, crowded into the frame with bindis stuck to our foreheads; my ballooned face grinning in triumph with my friend Helen as we met the sunrise on the summit of Mount Kenya; fourteen of us squeezed around the table at Christmas; my mum laughing on my dad's knee at a long-forgotten joke; a formal picture of my grandma and grandpa taken at church; one of Jeremy and I grinning at the camera from a trip that we took to the far north of Maine. Memories cemented by snapshots, a chronicle of highlights.

As I cleared my sheets of paper off the old dining table every night, I listened to my mum chopping vegetables in the kitchen. As I became attached to each voice, I could hear the ghost of my grandpa asking if I was sleeping okay and I could see the trace of his laughter lines in my dad's face as he urged me to take a break, to stop for dinner.

When I started to write the book I was wed to each of the interviews. In order to do justice to at least a handful of their stories, I started to write an oral history. I loved the beautiful irony of it, the idea of giving each person their fluent voice immortalized on the page. I spun myself between the interviews, slipping in pieces of my journey but wanting to be nothing more than a shadowy narrator.

As hidden as I thought I had made my own story, I was wary of showing the first draft to my parents. I watched them hover around the house as I wrote. I wanted their input, yet was nervous of exposing myself. Despite everything, I still wanted to hide my stutter from them, I still wanted to reassure them that I had a beautiful childhood, that my stutter was just a small part of me. I still wanted them to know that I was the strong, fearless daughter that they raised. My English upbringing balked against the frankness of my book.

However, I was high on stuttering in the aftermath of the NSA. As I returned to the origin of everything, I wanted to break the silence that I had always created around my stutter, I wanted to revisit some of the memories that surrounded me.

I began to transcribe one final interview that I had held in the LA home of film director and scriptwriter Barry Blaustein. As I typed I heard Barry and his wife Lorne talk about their son Corey, about their pain watching him struggle and feeling helpless. "As parents you go your whole life trying to put your children in the right atmosphere so they don't have a bad image of themselves, so they don't feel bad because of the stuttering," explained Lorne. In the space after her words Barry described how angry he felt at an awful teacher who had cut his son's lines in a school play because she didn't want to have her "masterpiece" ruined by his stutter.

It was easy to hear the pride they had in their son's empathy and his strength. But I could also hear how desperate they were to help him, how they wanted therapy to have all the answers. They remembered how he had been when he returned from the NSA, how he had become almost militant about his new mantra that it was okay to stutter, that he no longer had to try to be fluent. I watched how their smiles were tinged with nerves as they laughed it off. As Barry said, "It's very difficult to get him to talk about it."

His words felt eerily close to the bone. I could hear my parents in their voices, I could put myself in their son's shoes.

I could taste his burgeoning self-confidence, I could feel his determination to hold on to the feeling of self-acceptance that he had tasted at the conference. I could imagine his belief that only stutterers understood, that the fluent world could never fully comprehend his journey. I could feel the familiar alienation. I could vividly remember all the ways that my mum's insistence that I use my techniques had felt like criticism, all the times that I had shouted at her, all the ways that I had silenced the conversation.

Sitting in our dining room with my headphones on, I watched my mum in the kitchen. She was cooking while scribbling down a recipe and planning a tennis game. As always she was doing three things at once. As the recording of the interview clicked to a close, I watched her call down to my dad that supper was almost ready, I heard him slowly walk up the stairs from his office in the basement as she danced around the kitchen, plating everything up. I nodded as he silently asked if we should crack open a bottle of wine. Booze was a good idea.

I hummed to myself as I packed away my work and laid the table for three of us. Three plates, three glasses, as it always had been. I wished Jeremy was there, I wished I could feel his hand in mine. And yet I was glad that he wasn't. I wanted to have this conversation on our own. It was our history after all.

"Cheers, darlings."

We clinked our glasses together and then broke apart the sweet potatoes. Their steam billowed into the air between us.

"I was thinking . . ." What was I thinking? I hadn't planned how I would start this conversation. "I was thinking about the book and, as much as I want to have everyone's stories in there, I think I should change it. It will still have lots of their voices in it but, instead of straight oral histories, I think I want to write it as a memoir."

Until I said it out loud I hadn't decided. Yet, as cautious as I was, I knew that I needed to exorcise my own demons, that I need to write my own story. If I was going to ask all my interviewees to be so honest and vulnerable, then I had to be willing to do the same. However hesitant I was to write something so personal, I wanted to add a woman's voice to the male-dominated canon of stuttering literature. I believed that if I went public with my stuttering, I might be able to invite others to embrace whatever weakness they were dealing with.

"That's wonderful, darling." My dad beamed at me as he sawed into his steak.

I always knew that I had no bigger cheerleaders than my parents. Even Jeremy's life-sustaining optimism couldn't compete with their loyalty and their pom-pom shaking.

"Won't that be incredibly hard work?" My mum was always practical, always the one to ground my dad's heady idealism. She knew how hard I had worked at putting together the first draft.

"It will, but I think it is worth it. I hope anyway." She looked unconvinced so I tried a different tact. I steered towards logic and away from my personal motives. "I have pitched the book to agents and no one has been interested so far. There's no harm in trying something new, a new way of telling the same story."

I paused for a second. I couldn't skirt around the personal stuff forever. I wasn't sure how to broach the subject but I didn't have long. We were not a quiet family. I knew that my mum would leap in with a story of her own if I didn't pull together my thoughts quickly. "So, I have been thinking a lot about speech and growing up and how we all handled it. How rubbish I was at talking about my feelings, how I always got defensive when you brought it up. I realized I never really asked how *you* felt about it." It wasn't really a question, but I forced myself to stop talking and give them time to answer.

My dad chewed for a few seconds and then started speaking: "At first I wondered what was happening. It was the notable loss of self-confidence that really had me concerned. Your withdrawal and retreat into yourself scared me. It was like you had developed this self-protective shell that you retreated into. I was frightened that you wouldn't be able to get beyond it, that you wouldn't have a satisfying and fulfilling life. I remember watching you very closely."

He looked at my mum and carried on. "Gradually I saw you coming back into the real world, we both did. Somehow you had found the strength, the courage, maybe even the anger, to recover, to come back, to reassert yourself, and most of all to cope. Once I saw that happening, my fears started disappearing. I knew that you were going to handle it. Your life might be influenced by your stutter, but it wasn't going to be shattered by it. From that point on, I have never worried about you regarding your stuttering; it is to me just part of who you are."

I could feel myself tearing up.

My mum brushed his hand; she shook away the emotion

and leaned in. "I agree, but I worried about it. That was the difference between us. It bothered me because I could feel that you were not happy with the way things were for you. Luckily, you had great friends who supported you, but I know that you plowed through some difficult times. It is only as you have gotten older that you have taken on board what this means to you. Now it honestly doesn't matter. You have a fluid way of speaking; you demand that people listen to you."

She smiled as she said the last piece. I laughed with her. I knew that I had stubbornly demanded that people pay attention to me, that I had forced my way forward in spite of everything. I pushed my food around on my plate for a minute. "Were you ever embarrassed?"

There was not a second's pause: "Never." She had stopped eating. "I felt protective. I sometimes felt a degree of concern for the listener, I just hoped that they could handle it. I just hoped that they would appreciate you and wait. I think some people are just terribly ignorant. They really do not know how to handle a lot of things in life, and that is just another thing that they can't handle."

My dad was nodding his head. "I felt sorry for them. We could never be embarrassed by you. Plus we know that you are going to get through it. Come hell or high water, you are going to get it out."

I watched as my mum sipped her wine. She looked at my dad briefly and then said, "I think we took our lead from you. You were the one that was saying, 'This is tough but I can do it. Every so often I might need a little bit of help, but I can do it.' It was your strength that carried us."

She smiled at the end, a teary smile that made me lean my hand across the table and squeeze hers. Her hand felt small in mine, and I felt my dad lay his hand over ours. We sat there for a minute, grinning at each other and clinging on like three unglamorous musketeers. I whispered a thank-you and then asked my dad about his day at the office. As he started talking we moved off the loaded territory of my speech. I squeezed their hands for a final time. Unspoken as my words were, I wanted them to know that they were the ones who carried me, that they were the role models whom I looked up to all my life.

CHAPTER 11

LEARNING TO LET GO

New York, July 2011

THE LOFT IS teeming with bodies. The floor-to-ceiling windows at the far end are letting in whatever final rays of light can spill down the SoHo streets. I hear my high heels click along the concrete floor as I look around for some familiar faces. I don't recognize anyone. I'm rubbish at networking. I hate the surface-skimming chat and the eyes that are always looking over shoulders for the most influential person in the room. I would much rather be cradling a glass of wine and catching up with someone I cared about, but I had promised Jeremy that I would go. After a year filled with business plans and website designs, we have finally launched ExchangeMy Phone, our cell phone recycling and reuse business, a couple of months ago on a bootstrapped budget. I love the irony of it, the fact that we have turned the dreaded phone into a vehicle for good and created a business that celebrates the one piece of technology that we both grew up hating. I'm proud of all that we have achieved, but I'm well aware of its infancy. We have to get the word out there if we are going to keep making our rent payments.

We have been living in Brooklyn for half a year. After months of feeling broke and exhausted, I'm finally comfortable: the city now feels new enough to be an adventure and old enough to be home. Our tiny flat is starting to fill up with furniture, and friends are starting to crowd around the big wooden table that we had struggled to haul up the stairs.

We had moved to New York to be in the hearts of both the publishing world and the start-up tech community, and I'm quickly seeing what the latter means. It means exposed-brick offices, an average age of twenty-four, skinny jeans, oversized glasses, plaid shirts, and lace-up boots. It means hundreds of nerds and hipsters who have fallen out of the Ivy League and into the welcoming arms of angel investors. It means feeling achingly uncool. I'm not sure that my wardrobe is up to the job.

Tonight's party has been thrown by a heavily funded start-up, a company that wants to make it easy for everyone to learn anything from anyone. Months earlier I had stumbled on their website and signed up as a public speaking teacher. I had written the two-hour lesson plan, uploaded the description to their website, advertised the class, and fretted over who, if anyone, would turn up. It had not escaped my notice that each student had openly stared at me as I taught my first class. I had seen them glance at each other for explanations or reassurances as I started stuttering. Yet the class had gone better than expected. My years spent obsessively watching people speak had finally paid off. I knew a fair amount about the cadence of language and the power that could come from harnessing its rhythm, or trying to. I knew the strength of pausing, the excitement of a fast delivery, the nature of questions, and the beauty of storytelling. As I stood in the front of the classroom for the first time, I mentioned that I stuttered and joked I was a bit of an expert at it. Having led the class for more than an hour, I saw that my stutter had emboldened them. I watched in pride as each previously nervous student had stood up at the end to give an impromptu speech to the class. I suspected that, for all its negatives, stuttering had the impressive ability to break down walls, to put everyone's own fears to rest. If I could do it, they could do it, too.

As I squeeze towards the bar I finally see Danya's friendly face. She is behind tonight's bash and I slide over to congratulate her on the turnout. She's in her element, her face glowing as she chats to a couple and refills their glasses. "Hi, stranger," she calls out as we hug. She pushes her dark curls back from her face and pulls them up in a high bun. "Have you met these two amazing design folks?" I shake my head and she leans towards them. "This is Katherine, she's one of our best teachers."

They smile politely and I try awkwardly to brush off the compliment. I am still getting used to the heaping of praise that happens in America. She winks at me and then swings away to say hi to yet another guest, and I am left standing mutely in front of the two strangers. The woman shouts over the loud music towards me, "So what do you teach?"

As she asks the question her eyes scan the space just above my head. She's not even subtle about her disinterest. I can feel my chest contract instinctively. "I actually teach p p p p p p p p p p p p p p p p." I knew it would happen, but I'm still annoyed. I watch as her eyes slide quickly down towards me; I have captured her interest now. She exposes more of the white around her pupils as I carry on: "ppp p p ppp public speaking." I smile at the end. I hope it will erase her discomfort and mine. It feels like it works. Then she pipes up.

"Oh my gawd, that was so awkward." She laughs heartily. "You had me there for a moment but I get it now, p p p p public speaking. I get it. That's your shtick. That's the way you get everyone's attention. You make everyone feel super awkward, so they get that feeling of public speaking nerves, and then you speak normally again and tell them that you have all the answers."

Briefly I hate her. I hate her with every part of my shrunken body. I hate her lack of understanding, I hate her condescension, and I hate that she just ruthlessly mimicked me. I look at her partner. He's smiling but looks confused. I sense that he had not heard my quiet answer, but he has clearly not missed her braying.

Hatred burns itself out quickly and I'm left with the silence of deciding how to reply. Should I tell her that I stutter, that she is making herself look foolish and cruel? Should I walk away? Should I slap her? In the seconds that pass I play out every reaction in my head. As tempting as they may be, none of them are pretty.

Why do I care what this woman thinks of me? I remember something that the retired basketball player and sports announcer Bill Walton said to me as I sat in the tie-dye shrine of his San Diego sitting room: "You have to be less self-conscious about your stutter, you have to let it go."

I smile. Surprisingly, it is not the menacing, cruel smile that I would have once employed at a moment's notice. It may be traced with hurt, but it is a genuine smile. I realize that her opinion means little to me, that I'm not scared of the way she perceives me. However stupid her delivery, she's right. Stuttering can be awkward as shit, but not everything in life can be easy, not everything can be air-brushed to perfection.

"Actually, I st st st st st st stutter. I stutter every day, there is no speaking 'normally' for me. And y yes, I stutter when I teach. I'm a bizarre stuttering public speaking teacher." I pause for a few seconds, relishing the dumb look on her face. I'm not voluntary stuttering. Every block and repetition is viscerally real, but I don't mind. I'm enjoying it. I can feel the coolness of my British accent rumble beneath the high pitch of the room. "Surprisingly, you're rrrright though. Stuttering is my shtick, it is what I do best." I pause again. This time I turn and beam at her partner, "I h h h h h h heard rumors of a beer keg. Any idea where I might find that? I don't know about you, but I sure as h h h h hell need a drink."

· · ·

IN THE words of Jeff Blitz, "Stuttering can be terrible and funny at the same time and you don't need to pretend it's not." I'm not advocating that anyone should laugh at the spectacle of stuttering. There is something deeply cruel about anyone who laughs at someone else because they think less of them. But if we can laugh at the ridiculous situations that stuttering can trap us into, we should. Because laughter holds the potential to lessen all the painfully difficult situations. It can put them in the place that they deserve. Laughing together is far better than the awkward insult of an embarrassed shuffle. As much as I was always scared to hear the sound of a giggle in the wake of my speech, I was wrong. It turns out that humor holds us together much more strongly than it tears us apart.

Self-employed real estate appraiser Morgan Maxwell has a slew of stuttering jokes. My favorite is the one about a stuttering guy who wants to get a job as a Bible salesman. He interviews for the position, but the business owners are skeptical, "They say, 'Here's a dozen Bibles. Come back Friday afternoon and we'll see how you have done.' So the guy comes back six hours later and says, 'I've sold all the Bibles.' They are shocked, so they go with him the next day. They knock at the door of the first house and the guy says, 'Morning, sir, would you you you you like to b b b b b b b b b b b buy this b b b b b b b b b b b b b b b Bible from me now or w w w w w would you like me to read it to you?"

It's the truth behind Morgan's jokes that make them funny. I've missed innumerable trains because I couldn't say the name of my stop to the conductor. I've laughed at the overearnest politeness of two stutterers on the phone as we've sat in silence for long minutes, mistakenly assuming that the other was blocking. I've locked myself into the letter *f* enough times to recognize the familiar fear on my listener's face as they prepare themselves for what they assume is an oncoming stream of obscenities. I have collapsed into giggles as I've earnestly tried to tell people about a fabulous "ho ho ho ho ho ho ho ho ho hotel" that they really must try.

Before Bill Withers became the famous soul singer he is today, he worked as an airplane mechanic. When he left to pursue his dreams he still needed to make money, so he took a temporary job as a milkman. "This was 1965, I was gonna be the first black milkman ever in Santa Clara County," he remembers with a mischievous grin. "Some people wanted their milk put in their fridge, so I was given a key to their house. There were those who were just afraid of this big black guy and, instead of being able to put people at ease with my charm, I was stuttering and stomping my feet." He cracks up at the memory of their terror.

Telling jokes is a protection thing. If we can poke fun at ourselves, at all the awkward situations that our body gets us into, then we can stave off any other reaction. If we laugh the loudest we can drown out everyone else, if we lead the joke, then we can stop someone from frowning or looking away. As counterintuitive as it may seem, I tend to smile when I'm having difficultly with a word. I do it without thinking, but I expect it stems from a desire to put my listener at ease and remind myself not to be scared. I do it to acknowledge that something's happening, but it's not terrible, nothing to be afraid of or shocked by, nothing that needs to make them feel awkward. By smiling, I want to bring them in and give them the space to show their compassion. I agree wholeheartedly with the words of the actress Emily Blunt and her assertion that "More than anything, people are willing to see courage these days."

Bravery is not a choice for stutterers; you are courageous out of necessity. Every stutterer that I have ever met has been mocked at some point in their lives, everyone has watched someone walk away, everyone has seen someone frown or look at the floor. Everyone has heard someone's frustration or listened to them jump in and fill in their words. It is difficult to immunize yourself completely. However many times you see those reactions, however many times you tell yourself that they haven't killed you, you still see them. For much of my life, I assumed that my audience was at fault, that they should instinctively know how to react.

Today I sense that I always expected too much of them. I realize that I'm not at all sure that I would know how to respond if I didn't have a stutter, if I was in their shoes. My experiences interviewing other stutterers have taught me to be more circumspect with my judgment of others. I have seen what it means to watch someone else stutter. Today speech therapist Caryn Herring feels most comfortable around fellow stutterers, but she was not always so at ease, not always so comfortable in the role of listener. She remembers how scary she found her first NSA conference: "It was my first experience being around other people who stutter, and it made me uncomfortable. I wasn't sure where to look or what to do when talking to someone stuttering. After the first day or so, I became more comfortable being around them. Surprisingly quickly I began to envy the openness they portrayed with their stuttering."

In all honesty, stuttering is not an easy thing to behold, and there is no manual for our audience. We have all been educated in the most polite way to react to someone who has a limp or someone who is blind or someone using sign language. Yet, when it comes to stuttering, no one has been told what to do, no one has told everyone that there is a "right" way and a "wrong" way to react. I'm not all that surprised. It is not as simple as it should be. Not everyone wants the same reaction. Some stutterers like people to fill in their words if they get stuck; others can't imagine anything worse. The best our audience can do is to ask. But that requires a level of friendship and tact that is not present in every interaction. So we need to become our own ambassadors. As with any potentially awkward topic, we need to get over our own embarrassment and start talking about it. Jamie Rocchio is a good example. She makes sure that she thanks waitresses who are kind and patient, she makes sure to praise people when they do the right thing.

Is there one ideal reaction? As in everything, there is no definitive answer, everyone has their own opinions and preferences. Yet there are some standards that seem to be largely universal. As difficult as it may be, every stutterer will appreciate a listener who tries to see beyond the mask of stuttering, who reacts just as they would to anyone else. If you are one of those people who fills in everyone's words and cuts people's sentences short, don't stop on our account. Keep eye contact but don't make it a staring competition. Smile but not pity-ingly. Don't shut down the conversation, don't assume that we would rather sit in silence. Feel free to ask about the stut-ter, or don't. Oncology nurse Roisin McManus puts it best: "I want to feel that my listener wants me to keep coming to-wards them."

I have high expectations of my audience, I always have. And yet I have learnt not to be disappointed. I have learnt that my feelings do not have to be destabilized so easily, that my happiness is not dependent on any fluency that I may chance upon. I have learnt that being a "successful stutterer" is entirely on my own shoulders. As Jack Welch says, "It's the way I am. I have the view that this is the package you're get-ting. I hope you like it, or if you don't, there's not much I can do about it."

For much of my life I would have nodded in sage agree-ment and then I would have gone home and hoped that to-morrow I would be more fluent. I would have seen the term "successful stutterer" as a cruel oxymoron. Success would have meant finding fluency, somehow growing out of my speech and shedding my stutter like an unwanted skin. How-ever, it turns out that success is far more complex, far more hard earned, than that.

According to the writer David Shields, "Stuttering is like alcoholism: I will never outgrow it, and that's not my goal. In fact, I think I have conquered it by being very upfront about it. The beautiful paradox is that the more you are upfront about it, the less you stutter, the more relaxed the audience, so the more relaxed you become." David's idea subverts so much of what makes stuttering such a challenge. The dangerous cycle of stuttering follows that the more we stutter, the more nervous we become, the more our audience gets nervous and the more we lose any shred of control. The idea of instead building a self-perpetuating cycle of feeling relaxed and confident is deeply attractive, a difficult concept to take on board but a powerful one.

I have learnt to laugh at my stutter and to bring everyone else in on the joke. I have forced myself to speak in spite of it, to stutter on purpose, and to stutter openly. To send back an overcooked steak in a restaurant, to ask for exactly what I want, to pick up the phone and call back if someone hangs up on me—to be as fierce and silly and vulnerable as I choose to be. Above all else, I've learnt to keep moving forward. Jeff Blitz put it best when he told me, "I was not stopped or slowed down by my stutter. I was angry about it and sometimes ashamed, but I was never made small by it."

I have learnt not to wince when I hear the word *stutterer,* not to hear it as an insult or a swearword. Many of my friends in the stuttering world do not agree. They earnestly refuse to use the term, they prefer "person who stutters" or the more prosaic, "PWS." In comedian Rob Bloom's words, "I used to think of myself as a stutterer. Now I think of myself as a person who stutters. With a 'stutterer' that is all you are. I think that really defines you and limits you. It has a negative connotation to it for me. I have this image of a very, very low glass ceiling." On the other side, "A 'person who stutters' is like a 'person who has brown hair.' I like to say I'm a 'person who stutters' because it's just one part of me. It is just one small part of who I am."

I agree with Rob and appreciate the laudable sentiment behind his words. And yet I find the terms too professional, too clinical. I hate the idea of being reduced to an acronym on some speech therapist's notepad. Today I believe that we are free to call ourselves whatever we fancy. I choose to call myself a stutterer because I don't want to bleach out its power. I want it to be out in the open, and I want to face it directly, I want to erase the stigma of it. The word *stutterer* recalls unpleasant memories; it is loaded with prejudice and pain. Yet I believe that there is a certain power in subverting a word that I have long hated, something powerful in changing my own attitude towards myself as a stutterer.

Finally, I have learnt to understand that I will, in all likelihood, stutter for the rest of my life. It has not been easy. I have had to force myself not to be seduced by moments of temporary fluency. For years I would silently jump for joy when hours or days of fluency fell into my lap. Each time I would believe that this time it would stick around. My stutter was like some good-for-nothing husband who would be sweet for weeks on end and then come back to push me around. When he came back I would wish that he had never left, that I had never tasted fluency. Today I understand that they may, one day, find a cure. In the meantime, I have made myself realize that any lucky fluency I chance upon will not stick around. Like anything else unearned, it is flighty and not to be trusted.

Stuttering teases its hosts like no other disability. The blind are not periodically taunted with momentary sight, and the physically disabled cannot get up and stroll to the shops now and again. "Much of the time your speech may be uninterrupted, and then suddenly it is disabled for a moment," explains speech therapist Phil Schneider. "That creates a startle effect. It startles you and it startles the listener. Because we unconsciously have expectations, we think that the world is linear. We think that what you see is what you get, that the way you were yesterday is the way you'll be today." With stuttering nothing is quite so straightforward.

There are many people who seem to be fluent, who seem to have moved beyond their stutter. Yet, even those who have spoken smoothly for years still think of themselves as stutterers. Jake Steinfeld is a personal trainer and a motivational speaker. Although he makes his living using his voice, the possibility of blocking has never gone away, and even he can be taken by surprise. "I was live on the weekend *Today Show* on NBC," he remembers. "I was by myself and they had me sit in the greenroom for two hours before the show. I was just thinking too much." When the time came to appear on the show, "I literally couldn't speak. I said, 'I'm sorry, I don't know what's up.' I just got up and left. I just lost my mind. I got nervous. It was on NBC all over the country. But it came and went and it was done."

Jake talks about moving past the event, refusing to dwell on it. For much of my life I held on to my successes and failures far more rigidly than that. I lived in a neatly black-and-white world. Fluency meant success. Stuttering meant failure.

In my final year of university, my oldest friend Claire asked me to give a speech at her twenty-first. Her parents were jointly celebrating their wedding anniversary, so they had rented out the town hall to host the biggest party they could. Just under a hundred people were invited, and outfits were all that anyone discussed for months. Desperate to ignore my mounting panic, I didn't write the speech until the night before. By the time I was walking into the great hall I had memorized what I wanted to say but was visibly shaking. Claire whispered that I could ask someone else to do it, that there would be no shame in it. I grabbed Amey and asked her to stand by as my understudy. But the speech was so personal, full of stories and jokes that made sense only if I told them. So I gulped down one glass of champagne and watched as the speeches started. There was one before mine. I barely heard a word of it. Then I heard them call my name.

The flash of bulbs, the silence of the room, the stage looking out over the hall, hundreds of familiar eyes watching me. I began shakily. "Being asked to give a speech at your b b b bb best friend's twenty-first is a little bit like being asked to s s s s s s sleep with the queen. It's a great honor, but no one wants to do it." I stumbled over my words once or twice, but the opening joke got the laughter I had hoped for. The reaction propelled me forward. I leant closer in to the mic and felt the rumble of each word bounce back towards my lips. I blocked once on the next line and then I felt my voice slip into a rhythm. Ten minutes were over in a second. As I led the final toast to my "sister" and my adopted family, I watched as everyone stood with me. I walked down from the stage to the sound of clapping. Beaming faces rose to meet my own. I had succeeded. I hadn't made a fool of myself, and I hadn't ruined the night for either my parents or my friends. It was one of the best evenings of my life.

When the tape of the night's festivities arrived in the post, I ripped it open. My mum sat with me in our little den as I threw it into the video player with the present-ripping excitement of a child at Christmas. I listened to the interviews with the various partygoers in heady anticipation. When I saw my familiar purple dress alight on the stage, I sat back in my seat and smiled at my mum. I had never been excited to watch myself speak before. I had always refused to watch any tape that some well-meaning speech therapist ever made of my contorting face. But this time it was different—this time I knew that I would be looking at myself speaking largely fluently.

And yet there seemed to be something wrong. I had remembered that after my first few minors blocks I was fluent. Yet as I watched myself launch into my opening gambit, I didn't see the minor block I was expecting. I saw something breathy and anxious. Then I watched myself stumble some more. I ran my words into one another with my hands flying around my chest, trying to propel the words forward. My mum squeezed my hand. "Weren't you brilliant, darling." I wasn't so sure. That had been a good day, a great day in my mind. I couldn't help torturing myself with what I must have looked like on a bad day.

As ever, even my so-called successes were muddied by even the hint of a stutter. As ever, my failures and successes came and went but were not forgotten. Five years later, it felt like only a week had passed as I had taken the subway uptown through Manhattan.

• • •

I'M GOING to give a speech to a class of undergraduate speech therapists at Marymount College. The plan is to teach them about stuttering from the front line, to tell them the truth about stuttering from the proverbial horse's mouth. I have practiced my speech in front of Jeremy and recited my lines at least forty times in the peaceful quiet of our apartment. I know what I want to say. I know how I want to deliver my speech. Deep in my mind I know that they are expecting me to stutter, that they are coming to this class to learn. I know that I'm a walking, talking show-and-tell experience.

And yet I can't help it. A familiar voice in my head is telling me that I need to be fluent. I brush it aside and try to drown it out by silently repeating my lines as the subway jogs and stalls. The voice interjects. Do I know what a fool I will make of myself if I stutter uncontrollably?

I walk into the school and lean forward to introduce myself to the receptionist. I stutter like a champion. There's no chance that I'll suddenly become fluent when I give the speech. As I take the elevator up, I sigh. Come what may, the speech will go ahead. If I stutter on every word, then so be it. I will give them the best stuttering I can come up with.

When I finally stand behind the podium I'm calm, resigned, bathed in the adrenaline that I know will drown my fears. As I start to talk my stutter is nowhere to be found. It has somehow gotten stuck somewhere at the bottom of the elevator. I have no doubt that we will be reunited later, but I relish its absence. I feel powerful and eloquent and in control as I start to tell them some of my story, as I tell them what I would want from my ideal therapist. I'm having fun. I am so caught up in the thrill of it that I'm at least two paragraphs down when I notice how bored they look. As I start to tell them about a childhood grappling with stuttering, as I explain the fear and the deep scars the stuttering cut across my communication, I watch them doodle on their textbooks and stifle a couple of yawns.

"To this day I hate being alone, I hate silence. I am scared by the thought of sitting outside a conversation or staying home because I can't face my fear of introducing myself." I pause for dramatic effect. "It makes me feel like the stutter is winning and that I am being made invisible." I realize that my voice and my words are at odds, that they no longer reflect each other as neatly as they did when I assumed I would stutter.

Apparently it is more difficult than I imagined to convey the intricacies and challenges of stuttering, when my speech sounds surprisingly normal, when I sound like everyone else. Voluntary stuttering is the best solution I can come up with. I start throwing in some drawn-out, hard "fake" stutters. I repeat and push and block. I try to capture every stuttering trait I have ever seen or felt. I manage to capture their interest for a few moments, and then I lose them again. I suspect that they can see the voluntary stutters for the farce they are. The game is putting me further and further at ease, and any chance of a real stutter is falling further and further from my grasp. The class in front of me looks bored, disbelieving almost. I realize that they might think I'm a phony.

The class is kind enough; they don't boo or hiss. They ask questions and politely clap as I round off my speech. The teacher thanks me for my time and reassures me that her students have learnt a great deal from our afternoon together. I hope she's right, but I'm not so sure. As I leave the school I feel disappointed, let down. I realize that I'm not as effective without my stutter. I realize that, after years of trying to stifle it, stuttering is my message. I'm lost without it.

I realize that stuttering does not define me in the way I always worried it did, as someone to be pitied. I finally understand that, when everyone stood up to give a standing ovation at Claire's party, they were not clapping out of relief. They never saw my stutter as critically as I did; they had always seen beyond it. They had cheered because I had stuttered, because I had stood up anyway, because I had shown courage, because I was a good communicator in spite of my stutter, or perhaps because of it.

I never wanted to be vulnerable. I always believed that stuttering made me feeble because everyone could see my greatest weakness as soon as I opened my mouth. But it turns out that I was wrong. It seems that, for all of us, success and strength come from letting ourselves be seen with all our flaws and all our vulnerabilities. Our own success comes from believing that we are enough. As the research professor Brené Brown explained in her groundbreaking TED talk, "It appears that vulnerability is the birthplace of joy, of creativity, of belonging, of love."

There are so many myths that we tell ourselves, so much negativity that can be piled on top of our fraught speech. But there is one clear truth—our stutter, or whatever weakness we have, does not diminish us. Quite the opposite. Vulnerability draws people to us. We are attracted to people who don't have a façade up, people who are raw and unpolished. The people whom we want to spend our time around are the ones who laugh at themselves, the ones who are uncertain, the ones who can embrace those imperfect moments when they are recklessly human.

EPILOGUE

Brooklyn, August 2012

My story is not one of deliverance. I am not magically fixed as the curtain drops. Like an alcoholic who remembers the intoxicating taste of their late-night swigs or a manic depressive who remembers the sweet mania of their dangerous highs, my condition is not easily overcome. It is more than likely that I will know the experience of stuttering for the rest of my life. That I will forever taste the ghost of past stuttered words and feel the breathy delivery of the new.

And yet, after all these years, have I found the answers that I was hoping for? Have I reached some heady nirvana of total acceptance? I feel awkward shouting out a resounding yes. Because, in many ways, I am still the same person that I was at seven years old. In the twenty-one years that have passed since I started stuttering, my determination to conquer my stutter has not been rewarded, at least not in the way that I long hoped it would be. I still think about my speech, I still see the ways that people react to me, I still want to make my parents proud. Most important, I still stutter. To this day I am still not normal, whatever that means. I still stutter on my name and a million other words besides. I still have days when I would really quite like to order a sandwich without watching the waitress act as if I have morphed into some alien creature.

Stuttering does not have any neat answers. It is a messy condition full of gray areas. However, I'm better armed with understanding than I was before. I'm better aware of the profound need for change in the way we all perceive stuttering, in the way we all perceive normality. Having lived with the cyclic upheavals of stuttering, I am now better prepared to handle the roller coaster of my daily life. I am no longer seduced by moments or days of fluency. I know that my stutter is here to stay, that it will be my steady companion until I lie on my deathbed. Today I believe in laughing at my stutter, in addressing it and treating it with as much common sense as I can possibly muster.

In all honesty, I do have some of the answers that I was always searching for. I am a different person today. When I was growing up I saw my stutter as something that happened to me, something that held me back, something that marked me as different from the rest of the happily fluent world. I believed that if I were fluent, then everything else would simply fall into place.

I have learnt, finally, that happiness and fluency do not walk hand in hand as easily as I thought. It turns out that stutterers are not the only ones who have problems. It turns out that we all are in this messy, complicated world together, and the power that our vulnerabilities hold over us seems to rest on how we choose to address them. If you don't care, your problems don't really have a leg to stand on. If you decide to embrace them, they are totally dismembered.

I have often asked myself if, given the choice, I would swallow a magic pill and rid myself of my stutter. For much of my life I would not have thought twice about it. I would have overdosed greedily on whatever cure was offered. But today, the temptation is less appealing. Strange though it may sound, I choose to embrace my stutter. Four years ago I would have laughed at myself, guffawed at my foolishness. Today it is all a bit more complicated.

Stuttering takes away so much. It takes away the control that we want to have over our bodies, our appearance, and our language. It makes us small, it mocks us and teases us. It bleeds into every conversation and every relationship. The experience of stuttering is not fun. It is breathless and painful and scary. I would not wish my stutter on my worst enemy.

So why would I want anything to do with it? Because I do not know who I would be without my stutter. I have come to see that my stutter is me. It is not some dangerous devil on my shoulder, not some enemy that I am forever at war against. My stutter has made me who I am; I have achieved all I have not in spite of it, but because it. It might be the best thing that ever happened to me.

I have seen all of my flaws and my vulnerabilities lain across every room I have entered. I have witnessed the frailty and strength of my heart. It has made me humble; it has made me cry more violently and love more deeply; it has shown me the finest in people and the worst in them; it has made me sensitive to the world around me. In many ways my stutter is the best part of me. It has made me courageous and it has made me relish the every day moments that I have fought for. As Jeff Blitz neatly puts it, we should all "take genuine pleasure in those things that are not the gigantic victories but these little victories that accrue over the years."

I'm not sure who I would be without my stutter, but I can now appreciate the intensity my speech forces on my conversations, the perspective it has given me. I suspect that, without my speech, I would be less interesting to myself and to others. My stutter has ensured that, despite my height, despite my relatively "normal" appearance, I am not forgettable.

My stutter has shown me what it means to love, what it means to be loved, what it means to accept someone as intrinsically good. It has taught me to accept that we have all been designed to be, in the words of Phil Schneider, "perfectly imperfect." More than anything, I have seen that love can provide sustenance. It can protect us and push us forward. It can expose us to the beauty of every moment.

Love allowed me to write this book, it gave me the strength to change, to face the fear of change with as much strength as I could muster. My decision to leave England felt spontaneous at the time, but my choice to carry on, to see it through, not to grovel back to my job with my tail between my legs, was far more of a struggle. Change meant leaving behind a comfortable life in exchange for one that was far less certain, to abandon all my deep-rooted opinions about who I was, about who I could be, to be nostalgic for a time when I was less exposed and more guarded.

Growing up I was never one for dwelling on my own feelings, never keen on the thought of baring my soul to the world. As emotional as I have always been, I was always reserved in expressing the shifting tides of my moods. I always kept things behind closed doors and in the family. I forced myself not to focus on anything sad or painful for too long. Writing this book has helped me shun my long-fostered English reserve. Putting my life down on paper shattered the privacy that I had long sought to create. It may have been a catharsis that I wanted, one that I needed, but it scared me nevertheless.

What would people think of me? What effect would my immersion in stuttering have on my own speech or on the life ahead of me? Would dwelling on my stutter exacerbate it in some unforeseen way? Would my passionate resolutions stick with me in the years to come? Did I want to give up on the seductive notion that my stutter would magically disappear one day?

Luckily, my fears of what might happen were tempered by my fear of going back, of giving up all that writing had given me. Love fortified me and fear stopped me from leaning back, from looking over the edge. Whatever the reaction, I knew that honesty had to be better than the chest-clenching fear of hiding. I could no longer imagine the dreaded silence of stifling my stutter. I could no longer picture what it felt like not to be at the glorious whim of my unbridled emotions, to cry and laugh at the daily joys and conflicts of my life. Change had always scared me, but I could see how much it had given me, how necessary it had been for my life.

Today I can see that stuttering has given me far more than it ever took away. As I write this, I can hear Jeremy praising our employees on jobs well done. I can hear him talking on the phone to a customer and practicing what he'll say at an upcoming meeting. I know that he'll be exhausted when he finally crashes into bed at the end of the day. And yet I know he'll handle it. I know that we both will. Because coping with stuttering has hardwired a fighting instinct into us that has served us well over the years. Life is not easy, but we do not expect it to be. Writing a book, starting a business, and moving to a new country have been enormous challenges, but I know that we will make it work. Because we know that stopping, or giving up, or going back is never an option. We have learnt the necessity of moving forward regardless, of getting through whatever difficult moments arise and making ourselves heard. We know that the fight is worthwhile.

I left England wanting to escape, desperate to cure myself. Luckily, I found so much more than the meager scraps I was hoping for, something far more transformative. I explored my mind and learned to love both the body and the tribe that I was born into.

After years of coming to grips with a different kind of voice, with a different kind of life, I have learnt that it is our imperfections that ultimately make us beautiful. I have learnt that they are what give us our humanity and what bring us, finally, into focus.

ACKNOWLEDGMENTS

I FEEL INCREDIBLY LUCKY, and privileged, to be able to work with my editor, Sarah Branham. Along with Judith Curr, and the whole team at Atria, she took a chance on me and pushed me to make this the best book it could be. Sarah has been everything I could have wished for in an editor: deeply intelligent, thoughtful, funny, and unrelenting in her support. My literary agent, Brettne Bloom, has been a wonderful champion of the book from the first moment we were introduced. I'm grateful for her enthusiasm, warmth, tenacity, and perception.

In my year spent interviewing everyone for *Out With It* I was humbled by each person's generosity, eloquence, knowledge, and honesty. Hundreds of people responded to my phone calls, emails, and letters and told me their stories. I could not name every person in this book, but I am indebted to each of you. If it wasn't for you, this book would never have been created.

Thanks to Brooke and Morgan, my two favorite writers. Your perception, honesty, and writing expertise humbled me and inspired me to keep writing. I am grateful for your time, your wit, and your incredible cooking.

I am perpetually grateful to my friends. From Oman to Sri Lanka, Madagascar, Mexico, England, and America, I miss you all and often wish the world was a little smaller. I feel so lucky to have each of you in my life.

My debt to my parents is beyond words. They have loved me unconditionally in every moment of my life. They didn't just stand by me when I left my job to write this book. Instead they encouraged me and never let me believe that I'd made a mistake. They read every word, multiple times, looked up old diary entries, and answered hundreds of questions. I am in awe of their courage and always thankful for their laughter.

Finally, I can never adequately thank Jeremy, whose love is without reservation and whose faith in me is unfaltering, even when I am racked with doubt. During the years I wrote, and then tried to sell, this book he pushed me to clarify my thoughts, edited each draft, brought me endless cups of tea, and made my life wonderful.

RESOURCES

To FIND MY upcoming speaking engagements, read my blog, or explore further resources, please visit me at www.kather inepreston.com. The following organizations offer support, information, and services for people who stutter. For additional resources and a comprehensive list of stuttering organizations around the world, check out www.stutteringhomepage.com and http://www.isastutter.org.

National Stuttering Association (NSA): www.nsastutter.org
Information on stuttering, national support groups (chapters), and an annual US conference for stutterers, their families, and speech therapists. The NSA also publishes a quarterly magazine called *Letting Go*.

British Stammering Association (BSA): www.stammering.org
The BSA is the UK's national charity for both children and adults who stammer. Run by people who stammer, it provides information and support to all whose lives are affected by stammering throughout the UK.

Friends: The National Association of Young People Who Stutter: www.friendswhostutter.org

A volunteer organization created to provide a network of love and support for children and teenagers who stutter, their families, and the professionals who work with them. They host an annual three-day conference, regional one-day conferences, graduate and PhD training programs as well as teen-mentoring programs.

Our Time: www.ourtimestutter.org and www.campour time.org

Our Time is a nonprofit organization that helps young people who stutter improve their confidence and communication skills through arts programs, a summer camp, and speech therapy. The company offers its programming free of charge and provides financial aid for its speech therapy services and Camp Our Time.

StutterTalk: www.stuttertalk.com

A weekly podcast where the hosts talk openly about stuttering and interview people who stutter and leaders in speech-language pathology, self-help, and related fields. StutterTalk regularly reports from stuttering conferences and events.

American Speech-Language-Hearing Association (ASHA): www.asha.org

The professional, scientific, and credentialing association for more than 150,000 national and international members and affiliates who are audiologists, speech-language pathologists, and speech, language, and hearing scientists. ASHA's

Special Interest Group on Fluency and Fluency Disorders provides education, research, and support to help speech-language pathologists treat people who stutter.

Stuttering Foundation of America (SFA): www.stuttering help.org

Free online resources, services, and support to those who stutter and their families, as well as support for research into the causes of stuttering. Also offers extensive training programs on stuttering for professionals.

Stuttering Home Page: www.stutteringhomepage.com

Professor emerita from Minnesota State University, Mankato, Judith Maginnis Kuster (Department of Speech, Hearing and Rehabilitation Services) has a comprehensive site bursting with information, book lists, presentation papers, and more.

International Stuttering Association (ISA): www.isastutter .org

The international umbrella organization for stuttering associations. It produces the *One Voice* newsletter. Also its website includes a Bill of Rights and Responsibilities for people who stutter and links to stuttering newsletters from around the world.

Dominic Barker Trust: www.dominicbarkertrust.org.uk

A charity called Dom's Fund, set up to fund research into stammering.

The Stuttering Brain: thestutteringbrain.blogspot.com

A blog created by Dr. Tom Weidig, a theoretical physicist who now works in risk management, with a straight-talking approach to discussing the science, the treatments, and the controversies of stuttering.